MEDICAL TERMINOLOGY

Margaret L. May

Virginia Commonwealth University
Richmond, Virginia

MACMILLAN PUBLISHING COMPANY
NEW YORK
COLLIER MACMILLAN PUBLISHERS
LONDON

Macmillan Publishing Company
866 Third Avenue, New York, New York 10022

Collier Macmillan Canada, Inc.

Library of Congress Cataloging in Publication Data

May, Margaret L.
　　Medical terminology.
　　Bibliography: p.
　　Includes index.
　　1. Medicine—Terminology. 2. Medicine—Terminology—Problems, exercises, etc.
3. Anatomy—Terminology. 4. Anatomy—Terminology—Problems, exercises, etc.
5. Physiology—Terminology. 6. Physiology—Terminology—Problems, exercises, etc.
7. Pathology—Terminology. 8. Pathology—Terminology—Problems, exercises, etc.
I. Title. [DNLM: 1. NOMENCLATURE. W 15 M467m]
R123.M35 1985　　　　　　　　　610'.14　　　　　　　　　84.21451
ISBN 0-02-378293-5

PRINTING: 2　3　4　5　6　7　8　9　10　　　YEAR: 0　1　2　3

Contents

Preface

This text is designed to be used on a one-term undergraduate course for students who plan to enter the health science professions. Its purpose is to provide students with an etymological basis for understanding the anatomy, physiology, and pathology terms they will be required to learn in subsequent courses. It also could serve as a text for the professional development of employees of hospitals or for business people who deal with such areas as medical insurance. Although a classroom situation can greatly enhance this type of study, the book could easily be used by individuals who want to acquire this knowledge on their own.

A glance at the table of contents reveals that lesson titles follow an expected pattern. There are, however, a number of features unique to this text.

1. Most of the lessons include a list of related word elements and their meanings that students are responsible for learning.

2. Most of the lessons include lists of common names, illustrative words, or literal meanings. These items are included on the premise that the more associations students can make about meanings, the easier it will be for them to appreciate the rationale that produced the terms. Illustrative words are words that students are likely to know already; the fact that some are not medically oriented should point out that etymological study enriches our knowledge of language in general.

3. Lessons 23 and 24 deal with the many interesting ways in which medical terms have been derived other than from the basic Greek and Latin roots.

4. The lengthy review tests that follow Lessons 12 and 24 are organized to make the material relevant to anatomy and physiology courses. Review test 2 includes a list of frequently confused word elements.

5. The use of actual examples such as a medical report and a diagnostic checklist exposes students to some of the ways they can use their knowledge of words.

6. In addition to a large number of labeled illustrations with lessons on body systems, unlabeled drawings are included to reinforce anatomical knowledge.

7. Two crossword puzzles, one on the digestive system and one on respiration, follow their respective lessons. Solving these puzzles will reinforce students' learning of key terms.

8. Appendix A furnishes interested students with information about Greek and Latin.

The 24 lessons make the text flexible enough to be used for courses of varying numbers of weeks and class meetings. It can easily be covered by assigning two or three lessons per week during the term, allowing for an introductory class period and testing periods. Of necessity, lessons are not all the same length, a factor that can be taken into consideration in making assignments. Test material assumes that lessons are studied in sequence; however, Lessons 23 and 24 may be assigned at any time for extra reading or can be optional, and Lessons 11 and 13 may be assigned earlier if desired.

Acknowledgments

I appreciate the encouragement of the many students who have been involved in testing some of the lessons in class and those who expressed opinions about the format of the text and made many helpful comments about classroom procedures.

I also want to thank those who reviewed the manuscript, many of whom went over it with the proverbial fine-toothed comb, making constructive suggestions and catching my errors. Among those who offered helpful suggestions were Kathleen Kaiser, University of Missouri-Columbia; Robert Solomon, Essex Community College; Norma Walters, Auburn University; Burney Mendenhall, Kansas State University; Jeff Gliner, Colorado State University; Donald Peterson, St. Cloud State University; Judith Lynn Sebesta, University of South Dakota; Lou Stebbins, Louisiana Tech University; Yasmen Simonian, Weber State College; Jeannie Brock, Tarrant Junior College; Myron Fougeron, Kerney State College; Lois Knobeloch, Volunteer State Community College; Sandra Smith, Arkansas Tech University; Janet Bell Garber, Los Angeles Harbor College; Betty Jo Marshall, College of the Desert; Luis A. Losada, Lehman College; G. Nelson Greene, Delta College; Ruth Sween, Rochester Community College; Carol Seddon, Idaho State University; Harry Peery, Tompkins-Cortland Community College, and Janet Werner.

A word of thanks also is due to colleagues who loaned me reference volumes and to those persons who assisted in the acquisition of items for the Terminology Search exercises.

I would be most remiss if I did not mention the editors at Burgess Publishing Company. They offered their support, gave wise counsel, and kept me on my toes. The result is a stronger book than the one I had originally conceived.

To the Student

Students testify that a knowledge of terminology is of tremendous value in studying the health sciences. As a fringe benefit, it also enriches everyday vocabulary.

Experience has shown that you will need to spend one to two hours preparing for each class meeting. You will need to study the list of word elements and their definitions and take the self-test to indicate how well you have mastered the material. Repeat this procedure as many times as necessary to prepare for a quiz or test. For immediate reinforcement, check the answers at the back of the book. More attention is given to recognition of words than to word construction, for this is the way you will be dealing with these words in future courses.

At the end of each lesson there is space provided for you to record other terms that use the word elements presented in the lesson. Use this space both during class and when you read articles of medical interest. Doing so will provide additional reinforcement.

A glossary-index of all the word elements used in the book is included so you can quickly look up the meaning of one you have forgotten or a new one that you encounter. This index also indicates whether the term comes from Greek or Latin. Additional information regarding these languages is given in Appendix A. Appendix B lists a number of medical abbreviations.

This book is well illustrated. Labeled diagrams are included with each lesson on a body system. Pay careful attention to these labels, as they show how the word elements you are learning combine to form anatomical terms. Unlabeled illustrations, which appear with the self-tests, allow you to check your knowledge of anatomy. For additional information, consult an anatomy and physiology text or a medical dictionary.

At intervals throughout the book you will find a Terminology Search, an item of the type you will be expected to read in your future studies and during your career. These examples are included for your interest only unless your instructor makes assignments using them.

Comprehensive review tests are provided following Lessons 12 and 24. Use them to prepare for class tests. Throughout the course, you may wish to refer to the list of frequently confused word elements found as part of Review Test 2.

A medical dictionary will be invaluable to you during your career. You may want to purchase one to use in conjunction with this course. If not, a regular college level dictionary will be extremely useful for both definitions and pronunciations.

Note the P.S. after the last lesson, and remember to use the blank pages for listing additional word roots and terms as you run across them.

The study of words can be immensely fascinating; may you find it so!

LIST OF LABELED ILLUSTRATIONS

LIST OF UNLABELED ILLUSTRATIONS

Word Analysis

Analysis: from Greek, meaning dissolving

This is a course in etymology. The term *etymology* can be used to illustrate word construction.

etym- is a *word root* meaning true, literal.

-logy is a *suffix* meaning study of.

-o- is a *combining vowel* that links the word root and suffix.

Therefore, etymology means the study of the true, literal (meaning of words). Note that some part of the definition of a word may not be expressed but is simply read into the definition so it makes sense.

The suffix -logy illustrates another point about word construction. It is derived from:

-log-, a word root meaning study, from Greek (logos = word)

-y, a suffix meaning condition or process

These parts are used together so many times that the combination has become a suffix meaning the process of the study of.

Much of the terminology you will learn in this course is used in *anatomy*.

ana- is a *prefix* meaning in this case up or away from.

-tom- is a word root meaning cut.

-y is a suffix meaning _condition or process_
(See above if necessary.)

Therefore, anatomy means the process of cutting up or away from, which is what one has to do to learn structure (anatomy). Notice that no combining vowel is necessary in this word; can you tell why?

One of the current trends in medicine is the holistic approach. Hol- is from Greek (holos = complete, entire, total). An older, related term is *psychosomatic*.

psych- is a _word root_ meaning mind.
(See above if necessary.)

-o- is a _combining vowel_ .
(See above if necessary.)

psycho- is called a *combining form*, which is a word root plus a combining vowel.

somat- is a _____*word root*_____ meaning body.

-ic is a _____*suffix*_____ meaning pertaining to.

Therefore, psychosmatic means pertaining to mind and body, thus holistic; that is,[1] pertaining to the whole person.

Note that more than one word root may be used in a single term. You can find some terms in a medical dictionary that use five or six roots put together with *combining vowels*, of which -o- and -i- are the most common.

To review:

1. Words are built of elements called:

Prefix

Word root

Combining vowel $\Big\}$ which together are referred to as *combining form*

Suffix

2. Not all terms have all these parts.

3. The literal meaning may be shortened through usage.

4. Some parts of a definition may be understood without being expressed.

5. Elements sometimes are derived from a combination of shorter elements.

6. More than one word root may be used in a term.

Note: Did you observe that definitions of the analyzed words began with the meaning of the suffix?

TEST YOUR KNOWLEDGE

Analyze the following terms by writing the appropriate letter(s) under each element:

P = prefix

WR = word root

CV = combining vowel $\Big\}$ bracket as CF = combining form

S = suffix

(Meanings are given for your interest only; do not try to learn them now.)

For example:[2]

chondr o clast ic   pertaining to destruction of cartilage

WR CV WR S
$\underbrace{\text{WR CV}}_{\text{CF}}$

---

[1]Commonly written as i.e., from Latin (id est = that is).

[2]Commonly written as e.g., from Latin (exempli gratia = by way of example).

splen o megaly   enlargement of the spleen
WR CV S
  CF

peri card itis   inflammation around the heart

P   WR S   (Why is there no combining vowel?)

therm o graph ic   pertaining to record of heat
WR CV WR S
  CF

dys men o rrhea   painful menstrual flow
P WR CV WR S
   CF

cyst o scopy   examination of the bladder
WR CV S
  CF

phleb ectas ia   dilatation of a vein
WR WR S

pro gnosis   foreknowledge
P WR

lapar o tomy   incision into abdominal wall
WR CV S
  CF

blephar o plasty   surgical repair of eyelid
WR CV WR S
  CF

ather o scler osis   hard condition of arteries (due to plaque)
WR CV WR S
  CF

hepat itis   inflammation of liver
WR S

col o stomy   new opening into colon
P CV WR
   S

syn chondr osis   condition with one cartilage
P   WR   S

hem o phil ia   love of blood (predisposition to bleeding)
WR CV WR S
  CF

carcin o gen ic   producing cancer
WR CV WR S
  CF

angi o gram   record of a vessel
WR CV WR
   CF S

an esthes ia   without physical feeling

P WR S

hemi pleg ic   half paralyzed

P WR S

nephr o lith   kidney stone

WR CV WR S
CF

bin ocul ar   two eyed

P WR S

oste o por osis   condition of porous bone

WR CV WR S
CF

electr o cardi o gram   electrical record of heart

WR CV WR CV WR S
CF   CF

Answers to Lesson 1—page 207

4

Word Construction

Construction: from Latin, meaning to heap together

The emphasis in this book is on word recognition rather than word construction, but practice in building words reinforces knowledge about word elements. In this lesson you are asked to use the prefixes, suffixes, and word roots given to build terms that satisfy certain phrases. All these word parts will be included in future lessons; do not attempt to learn them now. Hint: If a combining vowel is needed, use -o-, which is correct for the majority of word roots. You will learn the exceptions in future lessons.

Prefixes		Word Roots		Suffixes	
a-, an-	without	enter-	intestine	-ia, -y	condition, process
dys-	bad, painful	(h)em-,	blood	-ic, -al	pertaining to
peri-	around	(h)emat-		-itis	inflammation
hypo-	less than, under	derm-,	skin	-osis	(abnormal) condition
post-	behind, after	dermat		-logy	study
endo-	inside	encephal-	brain	-ectomy	removal
		mast-	breast	-scope	instrument to
		hepat-	liver		examine
		card-	heart	-gram	record
		therm-	heat		

TEST YOUR KNOWLEDGE

1. Pertaining to under the skin _____hypodermic_____

2. Condition of bad intestine _____~~dysenterosis~~_____ _____dysentery_____

3. Condition of without blood _____ANEMIA_____

4. Study of the skin _dermatology_

5. Removal of the breast ~~encephalectomy~~   mastectomy

6. Inflammation of the skin _dermatitis_

7. Abnormal condition of the liver _hepatosis_

8. Pertaining to around the heart _pericardal_   pericardial

9. Pertaining to behind the liver _post hepatic_

10. Record of the heart _cardogram_   cardiogram

11. Condition of without a brain _anencephaly_

12. Pertaining to the intestine _enteric_

13. Study of the blood _hemology_   hematology

14. Instrument to examine inside _endoscope_

15. Inflammation of the breast _mastitis_

16. Inflammation inside the heart _endocarditis_

17. Record of heat _thermogram_

18. Inflammation of the brain _encephalitis_

Note: In the following phrases there is nothing in the definition to indicate a specific suffix. In cases like this, make a decision whether the term called for is a noun referring to a condition or a process, or an adjective pertaining to a structure. In most cases, nouns are given an -ia or -y suffix and adjectives are given an -ic or -al. For example:

-thermia or -thermy   condition of heat   _noun_

-thermal or -thermic   pertaining to heat   _Adjective_

You will gradually get a feel for which suffix is more commonly used. Meanwhile, consult your dictionary when necessary.

19. Around the breast _perimastic_

20. Under the heart _hypocardia c_

21. After the (partial) removal of the intestine _postenterectomy_

22. Without a breast _Amastia_

23. Inside the liver ~~endoenteral~~   endohepatic

24. Less than normal heat _hypothermia_

25. Bad liver _dyshepatic_

Now check your answers. If you made errors, analyze the reason you erred and make corrections.

Answers to Lesson 2—page 208

How To Use Lessons 3 Through 22

Lessons 3 through 22 have the same format. Each contains:

1. *A list of word elements and their meanings.* You will be responsible for learning these words and will be tested on them.

    a. In the Word Elements column, you will note the listing of two (in some cases, more) combining forms that have the same meaning. This occurs because many medical terms originate from both Greek and Latin, the dominant languages during the era of blossoming discoveries about the human body. Although you will not be required to distinguish which roots come from a particular language, note that when there are terms from both, the Greek term or terms will be listed first. Also, the appropriate designation of the language from which each word element originated appears in an alphabetical listing in the Glossary-Index that begins on page 245.

    b. Pronunciations are given where necessary. Prime accent is indicated by capital letters. To keep the number of diacritical marks to a minimum, only the long vowels are marked, as follows:

ā as in ray	ī as in light	ū as in cube
ē as in knee	ō as in cold	

    When word elements are combined to form a word, the accent and the letter sounds, or both, may change. Additional notes about pronunciation are given in Lesson 13. Meanwhile, listen to your instructor's pronunciation or consult a dictionary when in doubt about what is correct.

2. *Aids to learning.* In each lesson you will find columns of common names, literal meanings, illustrative words, or a combination of these, as is appropriate to the lesson. These columns, as their heading indicates, are *aids*; use them for this purpose only. The illustrative words may or may not relate to the health sciences. If they do, you will learn them in the course of working through the book. If they do not, they will help you appreciate the heritage of the English language and enrich your vocabulary. The derivations of words in the lesson titles

ILLUSTRATIONS

The illustrations included with six of the lessons give you a visual reference for many of the terms you are learning. In the labeled drawings, the words that you should know are in boldface type; pay special attention to these. To test your knowledge of anatomy at the end of the lesson, fill in the correct terms on the matching unlabeled illustrations following the self-tests.

TERMINOLOGY SEARCH

The adage, "Impression without expression leads to depression," points out the need to use your knowledge in a practical way. For this reason you will find, at intervals throughout the rest of the book, material that illustrates some of the ways you will encounter medical terminology in the "real world." These Terminology Search exercises follow Lessons 9, 12, 15, 17, 19, and 22. *You should not expect to know all the terms in any of the exercises,* but in reading through them you can expect to comprehend the material better than you could have without the knowledge you are acquiring from this course. When you have completed the book, read each Terminology Search again to appreciate your increased comprehension.

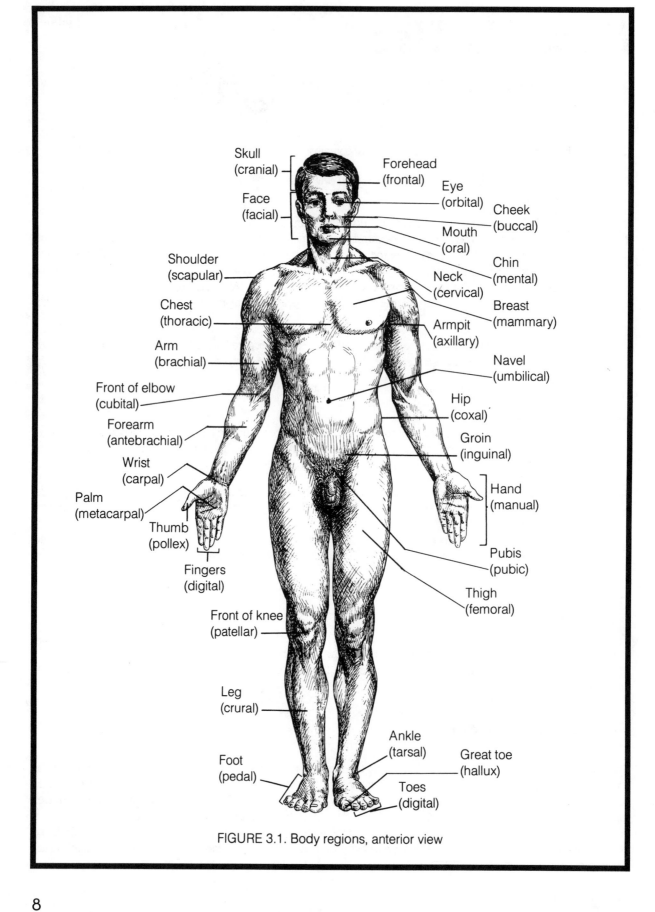

FIGURE 3.1. Body regions, anterior view

Body Regions

> **Region:** from Latin, meaning to rule

Read notes on how to use Lessons 3 through 22 before beginning this lesson.

Word Element	Anatomical Usage	Aids to Learning	
		Common Name	Illustrative Words
cephalo-, capito- **(SEF-a-lō)** **(KAP-i-tō)**	head		capital
rhino-, naso- **(RĪ-nō) (NĀ-zō)**	nose		rhinoceros, nasal
cheilo-, labio- **(KĪ-lō) (LĀ-bē-ō)**	lip		
bucco- **(BUK-kō)**	cheek		
mento- **(MEN-tō)**	chin		
auriculo- **(aw-RIK-ū-lō)**	ear		
ophthalmo-, oculo- **(of-THAL-mō)** **(OK-ū-lō)**	eye		ophthalmologist, binocular
cervico-, collo- **(SER-vi-kó) (KOL-ō)**	neck		collar
thoraco- **(THŌ-ra-kō)**	thorax	chest	

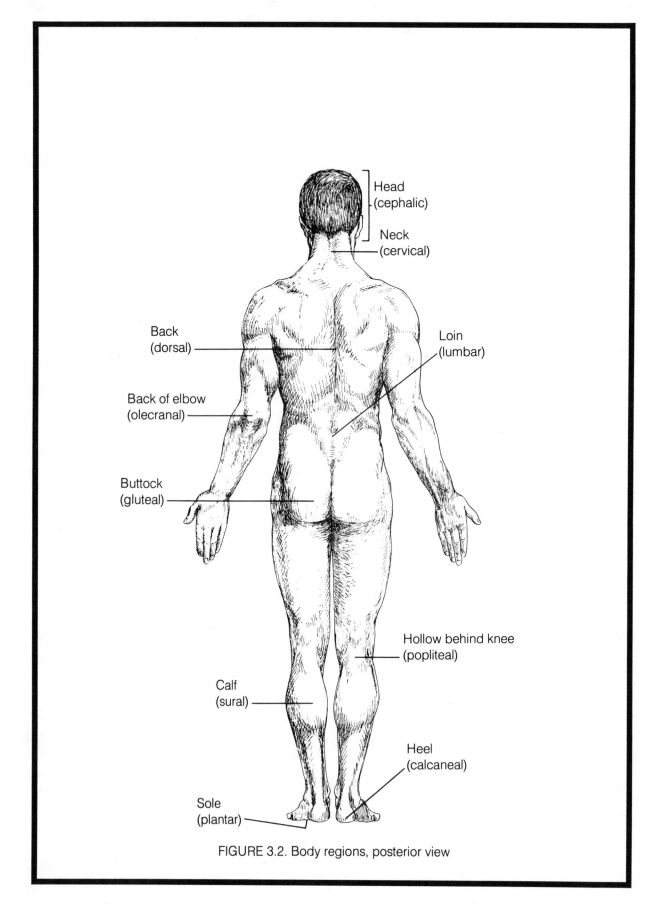

Head
(cephalic)

Neck
(cervical)

Back
(dorsal)

Loin
(lumbar)

Back of elbow
(olecranal)

Buttock
(gluteal)

Hollow behind knee
(popliteal)

Calf
(sural)

Heel
(calcaneal)

Sole
(plantar)

FIGURE 3.2. Body regions, posterior view

		Aids to Learning	
Word Element	**Anatomical Usage**	**Common Name**	**Illustrative Words**
stetho-, pectoro- **(STETH-ō)** **(PEK-tō-rō)**	chest		stethoscope, expectorate
masto-, mammo- **(MAS-tō) (MAM-ō)**	breast		mastectomy, mammal
thelo- **(THĒ-lō)**	nipple		
abdomino- **(ab-DOM-i-nō)**	abdomen	belly	
laparo- **(LAP-a-rō)**	abdominal wall	flank	
omphalo-, umbilico- **(OM-fa-lō)** **(um-BIL-i-kō)**	umbilicus	navel	
lumbo- **(LUM-bō)**	lumbar area	loin	
inguino- **(ING-gwi-nō)**	inguinal area	groin	
axilla **(ak-SIL-a)**	underarm	armpit	
brachio- **(BRĀK-ē-ō)**	brachium	upper arm	
olecrano-, cubito- **(ō-LEK-ran-ō)** **(KŪ-bi-tō)**	elbow		
antebachium **(an-te-BRĀ-kē-um)**	forearm		
carpo- **(KAR-pō)**	carpus	wrist	
chiro-, cheiro- manu- **(KĪ-rō) (MAN-ū)**	hand		chiropractor, manuscript
dactylo- **(DAK-ti-lō)**	digit	fingers and toes	

		Aids to Learning	
Word Element	Anatomical Usage	Common Name	Illustrative Words
onycho- (ON-i-kō)	nails		onyx
coxo- (KOK-sō)	hip		
gluteo- (GLOO-tē-ō)	rump	buttocks	
femoro- (FEM-ō-rō)	thigh		
genu- (JE-nū)	knee		genuflect
popliteal (pop-li-TĒ-al)	back of knee	ham	
cnemo-, crur- (NĒ-mō) (kroor)	leg		
tarso- (TAR-sō)	tarsus	ankle	
podo-, pedo- (PŌ-dō) (PĒ-dō)	foot		podiatrist, pedal
plantar (PLAN-tar)	sole of foot		plantar wart
parieto- (pa-RĪ-e-tō)	wall of body cavity		
splanchno-, viscero- (SPLANK-nō) (VIS-e-rō)	viscera	internal organs	visceral
coelo-, celo- (SĒ-lō)	coelom	body cavity	
dermo-, dermato-, (DER-mō) (der-MA-tō)			dermatologist
cutaneo-, (kū-TĂN-ē-ō)	skin		
integumento- (in-teg-ū-MEN-tō)			

WORDS USING THESE ELEMENTS

Record words given in class or encountered in your reading.

Word	Meaning
_____	_____
_____	_____
_____	_____
_____	_____
_____	_____
_____	_____
_____	_____
_____	_____
_____	_____
_____	_____
_____	_____
_____	_____

TEST YOUR KNOWLEDGE

Section A

Select the combining form that refers to each body part and write it in the blank.

1. Neck _cervico_   auriculo-

2. Underarm _axilla_   femoro-

3. Ear _auriculo_   dactylo-

4. Sole of foot _plantar_   parieto-

5. Digit _dactylo_   brachio-

6. Wall of body cavity _parieto_   cervico-

7. Wrist _carpo_   plantar

8. Upper arm _brachio_   axilla

9. Thigh _femoro_   thoraco-

10. Chest _thoraco_   carpo-

Write each term or combining form on the appropriate label line. You will not use all of the label lines.

Abdomino-   - Chiro-, cheiro-, manu-   Femoro-   Ophthalmo-, oculo-
Antebrachium   - Cheilo-, labio-   Genu-   Pedo-, podo-
Axilla   - Cnemo-, crur-   Inguino-   Rhino-, naso-
Brachio-   - Coxo-   Masto-, mammo-   Stetho-, pectoro-
Bucco-   - Cubito-   Mento-   Tarso-
Carpo-   Dactylo- (use twice)   Omphalo-, umbilico- Thelo-
Cervico-, collo-

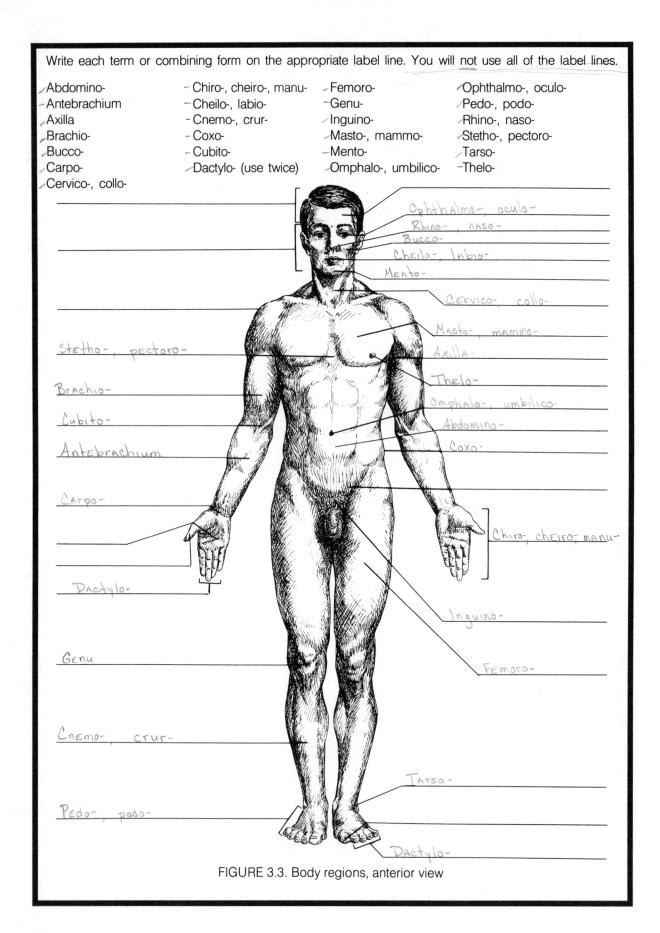

Ophthalmo-, oculo-
Rhino-, naso-
Bucco-
Cheilo-, labio-
Mento-
Cervico-, collo-
Masto-, mammo-
Axilla-
Thelo-
Omphalo-, umbilico-
Abdomino-
Coxo-
Stetho-, pectoro-
Brachio-
Cubito-
Antebrachium
Carpo-
Chiro, cheiro, manu-
Dactylo-
Inguino-
Femoro-
Genu
Cnemo-, crur-
Tarso-
Pedo-, podo-
Dactylo-

FIGURE 3.3. Body regions, anterior view

14

Section B

Select the combining form that refers to each body part and write it in the blank.

1. Forearm _antebrachium_   tarso-
2. Nails _onycho-_   cnemo-
3. Ankle _tarso-_   mento-
4. Groin _inguino-_   olecrano-
5. Chin _mento-_   carpo-
6. Elbow _olecrano-_   antebrachium
7. Hip _coxo-_   inguino-
8. Leg _cnemo-_   coxo-
9. Abdominal wall _laparo_   onycho-
10. Wrist _carpo-_   laparo-

Section C

Indicate to what body part each refers and give another combining form that refers to the same part.

1. Ophthalmo- _eye_   _oculo-_
2. Umbilico- _umbilicus (navel)_   _omphalo-_
3. Cheilo- _lip_   _labio-_
4. Capito- _head_   _cephalo-_
5. Splanchno- _viscera_   _viscero-_
6. Dermato- _skin_   _cutaneo-, dermo-, integumento-_
7. Pedo- _foot_   _podo-_
8. Pectoro- _chest_   _stetho-_
9. Masto- _breast_   _mammo-_
10. Rhino- _nose_   _naso-_

Section D

Give a combining form used for each of the following body parts.

1. Cheek _bucco_
2. Abdomen _abdomino_
3. Loin _lumbo-_
4. Hand _manu- cheiro- chiro-_
5. Nipple _thelo-_

Write each term or combining form on the appropriate label line. You will not use all of the label lines.

Auriculo-   Olecrano-
Cephalo-, capito- Onycho-   *nails*
Cervico-, collo   Plantar
Gluteo-   Popliteal
Lumbo-   Thoraco-

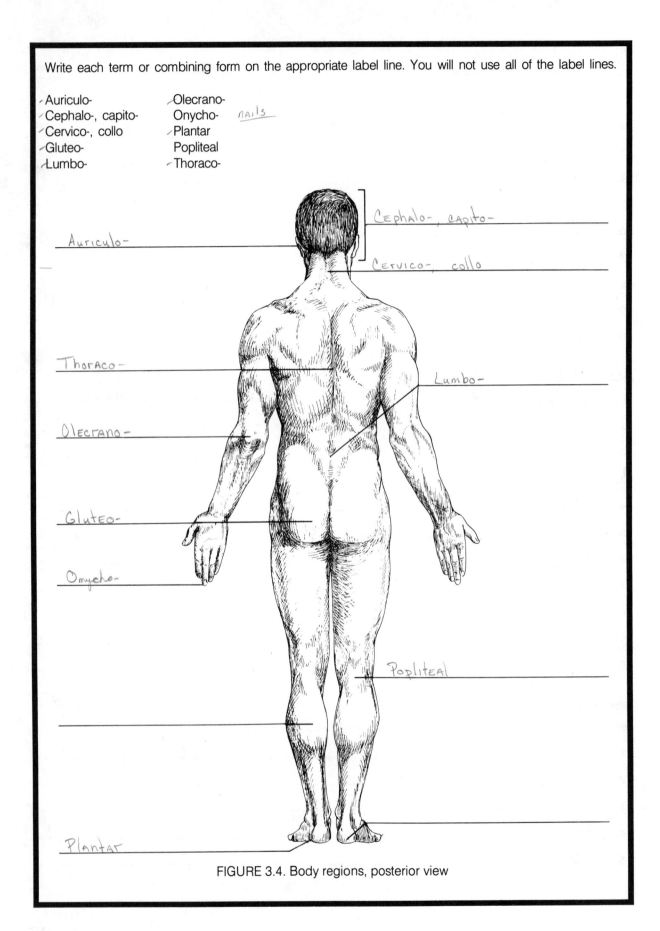

Cephalo-, capito-

Cervico-, collo

Auriculo-

Thoraco-

Lumbo-

Olecrano-

Gluteo-

Onycho-

Popliteal

Plantar

FIGURE 3.4. Body regions, posterior view

16

6. Upper arm _brachio-_

7. Buttock _gluteo-_

8. Knee _genu-_

9. Back of knee _popliteal_

10. Sole of foot _plantar_

Section E

Complete the following definitions.

1. Cephal/algia   pain in the ___head___

2. Ophthalm/o/logist   specialist in study of _eyes_

3. Steth/o/scope   instrument to examine the _chest_

4. Lapar/o/tomy   incision into the ___abdomen wall (flank)___

5. Hyper/dactyl/y   more than normal _digits (fingers or toes)_

6. Pector/alis major   large (muscle) of _chest_

7. Omphal/itis   inflammation of the ~~eye~~ _navel_

8. Bucc/al   pertaining to the _cheek_

9. Bin/ocul/ar   pertaining to two _eyes_

10. Mamm/ary   pertaining to the _breast_

Section F

Complete the following terms.

1. ___mast___ ectomy   removal of the breast

2. ___inguin___ ar   pertaining to the groin

3. ___abdomino___ centesis   puncture of the abdomen

4. Sub ___cutane___ ous   under the skin

5. ___onycho___ phagia   eating of the nails

6. ___pedo___ iatrist   healer of feet

7. _labio_ ___cheilo___ plasty   surgical repair of the lips

8. ___viscero___ megaly   enlargement of internal organs

9. ___dermato___ pathy   disease of the skin

10. ___coelo___ iac   pertaining to body cavity
        cel

Answers to Lesson 3—page 208

Suffixes

> **Suffix:** from Latin, meaning fasten under. (The b of the Latin sub, meaning under, is softened to f.)

Notice as you study these suffixes that some of them are really compounds of a word root and a suffix (e.g., -tomy is composed of tom meaning cut and y meaning condition; -genic is composed of gen meaning produce and -ic meaning pertaining to). Purists would insist on making these separations, but the total suffixes are presented in this book, as is the practice in medical dictionaries.

You will encounter some terms that have two suffixes (e.g., biolog/ic/al, psycholog/ic/al).

		Aids to Learning	
Suffix	**Meaning**	**Illustrative Words**	**Literal Meaning**
-al, -ic, -ous, -ac, -eal,-ar -ary, -ory	pertaining to	electric, thermal, mucous, auditory	
-ase	enzyme		
-clast	break down		
-ectomy (EK-tō-mē)	excision, removal	appendectomy	cut out
-ectasia (ek-TĀ-zē-a)	dilatation		stretch out
-genesis	production, formation		
-genic	producing, forming	carcinogenic	
-graph	instrument to record	cardiograph	
-graphy	recording	stenography	

Suffix	Meaning	Illustrative Words	Literal Meaning
-gram	record of	cardiogram	
-ia, -y	condition, process	hypoglycemia, diathermy	
-ist	specialist	dentist	
-itis	inflammation	laryngitis	
-logy	study of	biology	
-logist	specialist in the study of	psychologist	
-lysis (LĪ-sis)	decomposition, destruction	analysis	
-meter	instrument to measure	thermometer	
-metry	measurement	geometry	
-megaly (ME-ga-lē)	enlargement		
-oid	resembling	cuboid, spheroid	
-ose, -ous	full of	verbose, gracious	
-osis, -iasis, -ism	condition (often abnormal)	halitosis, hypothyroidism	
-penia (PĒ-nē-a)	deficiency		
-plasia (PLĀ-zē-a)	formation (often abnormal)	neoplasia, plastic	
-plasty	repair		
-poiesis (poi-Ē-sis)	formation (usually on a continuing basis)		
-rrhea (RĒ-a)	flow	diarrhea	
-scope	instrument to examine	stethoscope	
-scopy	examination	microscopy	
-stenosis (ste-NŌ-sis)	constriction, narrowing		

Suffix	Meaning	Illustrative Words	Literal Meaning
-stomy	formation of new opening	colostomy	process of mouth
-tomy	incision	tracheotomy	process of cutting
-tripsy	crushing, friction		

WORDS USING THESE ELEMENTS

Record words given in class or encountered in your reading.

Word	Meaning
_____	_____
_____	_____
_____	_____
_____	_____
_____	_____
_____	_____
_____	_____
_____	_____
_____	_____
_____	_____
_____	_____

TEST YOUR KNOWLEDGE

Section A

Select the suffix that has the meaning given and write it in the blank. Then think of a word that uses the suffix and record it.

-logy	-oid
-itis	-meter
-genic	-ic, -al
-osis, -ia	-scopy
-ectomy	-clast

		Suffix	Example
1.	Excision	-ectomy	tonselectomy
2.	Inflammation	-itis	
3.	Resembling	-oid	sigmoid
4.	Examination	-scopy	
5.	Break down	-clast	
6.	Pertaining to	-ic, -al	
7.	Producing	-genesis	
8.	Study	-logy	biology
9.	Condition	-osis, -ia	
10.	Instrument to measure	-meter	

Section B

Select the suffix that has the meaning given and write it in the blank. Then think of a word that uses the suffix and record it.

-penia	-lysis
-tomy	-stomy
-stenosis	-gram
-megaly	-ist
-ectasia	-rrhea

		Suffix	Example
1.	Record	-gram	cardiogram
2.	Decomposition	-lysis	photolysis
3.	Deficiency	-penia	leukopenia
4.	Formation of new opening	-stomy	colostomy
5.	Incision	-tomy	
6.	Enlargement	-megaly	

22

7. Flow ___-rrhEA___ ___diArrhEA___

8. Constriction ___-stEnosis___ _____

9. Specialist ___-ist___ ___psychologist___

10. Dilatation ___-EctAsiA___ _____

Section C

List all the suffixes that have the following meanings.

1. Formation ___poESis___ ___plAsiA___ ___gEnEsis___

2. Pertaining to ___ic, Al, EAl,___ ___ous, Ac, Ar,___ ___Ary, ory___

3. Condition ___osis___ ___iAsis___ ___ism___ ___iA___ ___y___

4. Process ___iA___ ___y___

Section D

Write in the meaning of

1. -ase ___EnzymE___

2. -ose ___Full of___

3. -clast ___brEAk down___

4. -graph ___record of___ ___instrumEnt to rEcord___

5. -logist ___spEciAlist in thE study of___

6. -scope ___instrumEnt to EXAminE___

7. -tripsy ___crushing___

Section E

Following is a list of terms constructed by using combining forms from Lesson 3 and suffixes from this lesson. Using slash marks, divide these into word elements and define the whole term.

1. Mastoid ___rEsEmbEling A brEAst___

2. Stethoscope ___instrumEnt to EXAminE thE chEst___

3. Rhinitis ___inflAmmAtion of thE nosE___

4. Mammogram ___rEcord of thE brEAst___

5. Laparotomy ___incision in thE AbdominAl wAll___

6. Ophthalmology ___study of thE EyE___

7. Chiropodist ___spEciAlist of thE hAnd And foot___

8. Cephalic ___pErtAining to thE hEAd___

9. Onychosis ___condition of thE nAils___

10. Cutaneous ___pErtAining to thE skin___

Section F

Complete the following definitions.

1. Oo/genesis _____ Production _____ *Formation* _____ of eggs
2. Electr/o/cardi/o/gram electrical _____ record _____ of the heart
3. Lip/oid _____ resembeling _____ fat
4. Gastr/o/scopy _____ examination _____ of the stomach
5. Pelvi/metry _____ measurement _____ of the pelvis
6. Hypo/plasia less than normal ~~growth~~ FORMATION _____
7. Mitral stenosis _____ CONSTRICTION _____ of the mitral (valve of the heart)
8. Oste/o/clast _____ break down _____ of bone
9. A/men/o/rrhea without menstrual _____ flow _____
10. Hemat/o/poiesis _____ formation ~~deficiency~~ _____ of blood (cells)

Section G

Complete the following terms.

1. Bronchi ectasia _____ dilation of the bronchi
2. Splen/o megaly _____ enlargement of the spleen
3. Cyst/o ~~gram~~ graphy _____ recording of the bladder
4. Gynec/o logist _____ specialist in the study of women
5. Hem/o lysis _____ destruction of blood
6. Lith/o tomy _____ incision (to remove) a stone
7. Erythr/o ~~poeisis~~ penic *formation* _____ deficiency of red (blood cells)
8. Path/o genic _____ producing disease
9. Cardi/o megaly _____ enlargement of the heart
10. Angi/o tripsy _____ crushing of a vessel

no way tomy graphy

Answers to Lesson 4—page 210

24

Normal Body Processes

Normal: from Latin, meaning according to pattern
Process: from Latin, meaning going before

Word Element	Meaning	Aids to Learning	
		Illustrative Words	**Literal Meaning**
bio-	living	biology	
-kinesia (ki-NĒ-sē-a)	movement	kinesiology	
mento-	thinking	mental	
-phasia (FĀ-zē-a)	speech		
-phoria (FŌ-rē-a)	emotional feeling	euphoria	
somni-, dormi-	sleeping	insomnia, dormitory	
-esthesia (es-THĒ-zē-a)	physical sensation	anesthesia	
opto-, optico-, -opsy, -opia (Ō-pē-a)	vision	optical, biopsy	
acousto-, audito- (a-KOOS-tō) (AW-di-tō)	hearing	acoustic, auditory	
olfacto-, -osmia (ol-FAK-tō) (OZ-mē-a)	smell	olfactory	

Word Element	Meaning	Illustrative Words	Literal Meaning
gusto-, -geusia (GŪ-zē-a)	taste	gustatory, disgust	
-aphia, tacto- (Ā-fē-a)	touch	tactful, tactile	
-pnea, spiro- (NĒ-a) (SPĪ-rō)	breathing	apnea, inspiration	
-orexia (ō-REK-sē-a)	appetite	anorexia	
dipso-, -dipsia	thirst	dipsomaniac	
mastico- (MAS-ti-kō)	chewing	masticate	
phago-, -phagia (FAG-ō) (FĀ-jē-a)	eating, swallowing		
-pepsia (PEP-sē-a)	digestion	dyspepsia	digest = carry apart
defeca- (DEF-e-ka)	elimination of feces	defecation	
urino- (Ū-ri-nō)	urination		
meno-	menstruation	menopause	month
-cyesis, gest- (si-Ē-sis) (jest)	pregnancy	gestation	gest = carry
-par-	giving birth		
-physis (FĪ-sis)	growth		
-crin-	secretion	endocrine	secrete
peristalsis (per-i-STAL-sis)	muscle contraction in internal organs		contract around

WORDS USING THESE ELEMENTS

Record words given in class or encountered in your reading.

Word	Meaning

TEST YOUR KNOWLEDGE

Section A

Give the meaning of the following combining forms and then give the suffix that has the same meaning.

		Meaning	Suffix
1.	Phago-	EAting	-phagia
2.	Gusto-	taste	-geusia
3.	Gest-	pregnancy	-cyesis
4.	Olfacto-	smell	-osmia
5.	Opto-	vision	-opty
6.	Tacto-	touch	-aphia
7.	Spiro-	breathing	-pnea

Section B   ic ac ar ary ory eal ous al

The following terms add suffixes from Lesson 4 to combining forms from this lesson. Using slash marks, divide these terms into word elements and then define the whole term.

1. Olfactory _pertaining to smell_
2. Optic _pertaining to vision_
3. Auditory _pertaining to hearing_

27

4. Acoustic _pertaining to hearing_

5. Biology _study of living (organisms)_

6. Mental _pertaining to the mind thinking_

7. Gustatory _pertaining to taste_

8. Spirometer _instrument to measure breathing_

9. Menorrhea _menstrual flow_

10. Urinary _pertaining to the (condition of the urine)_
    urine
    ↓
    - urea

Section C

Write in the word element from the list that is indicated by each definition. Then give a word you know that uses each.

-orexia	-pepsia
somni-	phasia
mastico-	dipso-
crin-	-esthesia
-phoria	

		Element	**Example**
1.	Emotional feeling	-phoria	Euphoria
2.	Physical sensation	-esthesia	Anesthesia
3.	Appetite	-orexia	Anorexia
4.	Digestion	-pepsia	
5.	Secretion	crin-	Endocrin gland
6.	Speech	phasia	dysphasia ?
7.	Sleeping	somni-	insomnia
8.	Chewing	mastico-	
9.	Thirst	dipso-	

Section D

Define the following.

1. -kinesia _movement_

2. -aphia _TOUCH_

3. -pnea _deficiency_ _BREATHING_

4. Phago- _Eating_

5. Defeca- _Elimination of feces_

28

6. Urino- _urination_

7. Paro- _GIVING BIRTH_

8. -physis _GROWTH_

9. Peristalsis _muscle contraction of internal organs_

Section E

Complete the following definitions.

1. Dys/geusia   bad _taste_

2. Kin/esthesia   _physical sensation_ of movement

3. Hypo/physis   _GROW_ under

4. Endo/crine   _secretion_ within

5. Poly/dipsia   much _thirst_

6. Spiro/meter   instrument to measure _breathing_

7. Bi/opsy   _VISION_ ~~removal~~ of living (tissue)

8. Hyper/pnea   more than normal _BREATHING_

9. A/phasia   without _SPEECH_

10. Nulli/para   (woman who has) not _GIVEN BIRTH_

Section F

Complete the following definitions.

1. An _orexia_   without appetite

2. Eu _phoria_   good emotional feeling

3. Pseudo _cyesis_   false pregnancy

4. _meno_ rrhagia   excessive menstrual flow

5. _phago_ cyte   cell that eats

6. Vivi _par_ ous   giving birth to living (young)

7. Pro _gest_ erone   (hormone) for (in favor of) pregnancy

8. _Audit_ ory   pertaining to hearing

9. _mastic_ ation   process of chewing

10. _SOMN_ ambulism   sleep-walking

Answers to Lesson 5—page 212

Prefixes

Prefix: from Latin, meaning fasten before

As is true of suffixes, some prefixes are properly word roots that are used so often at the beginning of a word that they have come to be known as prefixes. Some of these word roots are found in suffixes as well as in prefixes (e.g., megalo/cardia and cardio/megaly both mean enlarged heart; cardiomegaly is the preferred term).

You will sometimes encounter prefixes in the middle of a term (e.g., my/a/sthenia means without muscle strength; -asthenia is used as a suffix denoting weakness). In neuro/hypo/physis, hypo- is an integral part of hypophysis, another name for the pituitary gland, and neuro- (nerve) indicates a certain part of the gland.

Prefix	Meaning	Illustrative Words
a-, an-	without	atonal, anesthetic
ad-	toward	adhere
ana-	up	anatomy
ante-	before	antecedent
anti-, contra-	against	antiseptic, contraceptive
apo-	from	apogee
auto-	self	automatic
cata-	down	catastrophe
dia-, per-	through	diarrhea, perforation
dis-	apart	disjointed
dys-	bad, difficult, painful	dysentery
ecto-	outside	ectoplasm
en-	in	entangle
endo-, ento-	inside	endocrine
epi-	upon	epidermis
eu-	good, normal, healthy	euphoria

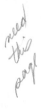

Prefix	Meaning	Illustrative Words
ex-, exo-	out, away	external, exotic
extra-	more than, outside of	extrasensory
hemi-, semi-	half	hemisphere, semicircular
homeo-	similar	homeostasis
homo-, iso-	same	homosexual, isobar
hetero-	different, other	heterogeneous
hypo-	under, less than normal	hypodermic, hypoglycemia
hyper-	more than normal	hypertension, hyperactive
in-	into, not	inoculate, insensitive
infra-, sub-	below	infrared, submarine
inter-	between	interpersonal
intra-	within	intramural
macro-, megalo-	large	macroscopic, megalopolis
mal-	bad	malaria
meta-	beyond (in degree or position)	metatarsal, metabolism
micro-	small	microorganism
neo-	new	neonatal
para-	beside, beyond, abnormal	paranoid, paralysis
peri-, circum-	around	perimeter, circumstance
poly-	many, much	polygamy
post-, retro-	behind, after	postoperative, retroactive
pro-, pre-	in front of, before	prognosis, premolar
semi-	partly	semisolid
supra-, super-	above, more than	suprarenal, supersaturated
syn-, con-	with, together	syndrome, conjunctiva
trans-	across, through	transcontinental

32

WORDS USING THESE PREFIXES

Record words given in class or encountered in your reading.

Word	Meaning

TEST YOUR KNOWLEDGE

Section A

Select from the list the prefix used for each definition given. Then write in a word you know that uses it.

micro-   neo-
eu-   hyper-
epi-   auto-
intra-   post-
trans-   ante-

		Prefix	**Example**
1.	More than normal	hyper-	hypersensitive
2.	Within	intra-	intramolecular
3.	Small	micro-	
4.	Before	Ante-	Antecedent
5.	Upon	Epi-	
6.	Across	trans-	transfusion
7.	New	neo-	neonatal
8.	Behind	post-	post traumatic
9.	Good	eu-	Euphoria
10.	Self	Auto-	Autolysis

Section B

For each prefix given write the meaning. Then give another prefix that means the same thing.

1. Megalo- _enlargement_   MACRO   _____
2. Con- _~~against~~ with, together_   SYN   _~~convert~~ congregation_
3. Iso- _same_   HOMO   _isometric_
4. Hemi- _half_   SEMI   _hemisphere_
5. Peri- _around_   CIRCUM   _____
6. Anti- _against_   CONTRA   _antiparallel_
7. Infra- _below_   HYPO   _____

Section C

The following terms combine prefixes with the combining forms in Lesson 5. Using slash marks, divide these terms into word elements and then define the whole term.

check

1. Apnea _without breathing_
2. Dyspepsia _painful (bad) digestion_
3. Euphoria _good emotional feeling_
4. Hyperesthesia _more than normal (dilation = ectasia) physical sensation_
5. Endocrine _secretion within_
6. Diaphysis _+) growth_
7. Anaphia _without touch_

Section D

Divide and define the following terms, which are constructed from word elements in Lessons 1 through 6.

1. Postnasal _(After) PERTAINING TO behind the nose_
2. Chiropodist _specialist of hands & feet_ hand ft.
3. Neoplasia _new formation_
4. Spirometer _instrument to measure breathing_
5. Perimastitis _inflammation around the breast_
6. Axillary _pertaining to the armpit_
7. Dermatologist _specialist in the study of the skin_
8. Subcutaneous _pertaining to UNDER below the skin_
9. Pneumograph _INSTRUMENT TO record of breathing_
10. Hypodermic _pertaining to under the skin_
11. Cephalic _pertaining to the head_
12. Polydactyly _condition of many digits (fingers/toes)_

34

13. Auricular *pertaining to the external ear*

14. Dysmenorrhea *bad menstrual flow*

15. Visceral *pertaining to the viscera (internal organs)*

Section E

al ic ac ous ory ary eal ar

Complete the following definitions.

1. Ante/nat/al   *pertaining to before*   birth

2. Hemi/plegia   *partial*   paralysis

3. Hypo/plasia   *less than normal*   formation

4. Trans/derm/al   *pertaining to across (through)*   the skin

5. Poly/mast/ia   *many conditions of the*   breasts

6. Inter/cost/al   *pertaining to between*   the ribs

7. Iso/ton/ic   *pertaining to the same*   tone

8. Retro/periton/eal   *pertaining to behind*   the peritoneum

9. Per/or/al   the mouth

10. Anti/sepsis   *against*   infecton

Section F

Complete the following terms.

1. *dys* entery   bad digestion

2. *Epi* dermis   upon the skin

3. *Intra* cellular   within the cell

4. *micro* scopy   examination of small things

5. renal   above the kidney *supra*

6. *CONTRA~~Anti~~* ception   against fertilization

7. *A~~s~~* sthenia   without strength

8. *Auto* immune   immune reaction to self

9. *PRE* molar   in front of molar (teeth)

10. *hyper* emia   more than normal blood

Note: From this point on, practice exercises will make use of the material from Lessons 1 through 6. Review these lessons whenever necessary.

Answers to Lesson 6—page 214

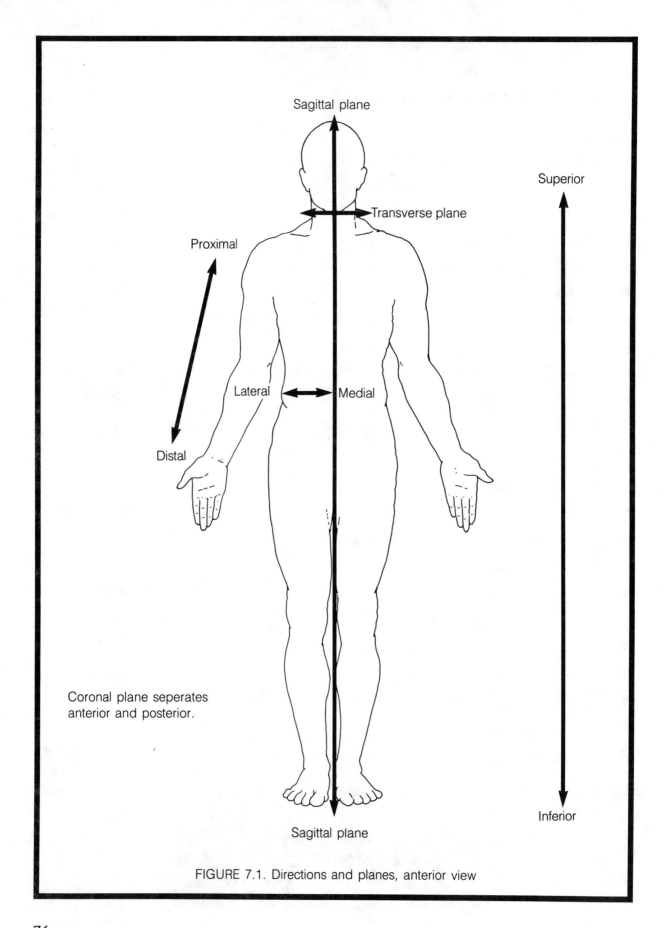

Coronal plane seperates anterior and posterior.

FIGURE 7.1. Directions and planes, anterior view

Directions and Planes

> **Direction:** from Latin, meaning to make straight
> **Plane:** from Latin, meaning level, flat

In an anatomy course the terms given in this lesson are used for at least two basic purposes: (1) to refer in descriptive writing to the spatial relationship of one body part to another and (2) to interpret illustrations of sections of body parts.

  The reference point for all these terms is anatomical position (i.e., erect posture with palms to the front).

		Aids to Learning	
Term	**Anatomical Use**	**Illustrative Words**	**Literal Meaning**
		Directions	
posterior, dorsal (pos-TĒ-rē-or) (DOR-sal)	back		dorsum = the back post = after
anterior, ventral (an-TĒ-rē-or) (VEN-tral)	front		ventr = belly ante = before
lateral (LAT-er-al)	side	unilateral	
medial, mesial (MĒ-dē-al) (MĒ-zē-al)	middle	medium, intermediate	
proximal (PROK-si-mal)	near to*	approximate	
distal (DIS-tal)	far from*	distant	

* (e.g., as parts of appendages relate to trunk, blood vessels to heart, and nerves to brain or spinal cord.)

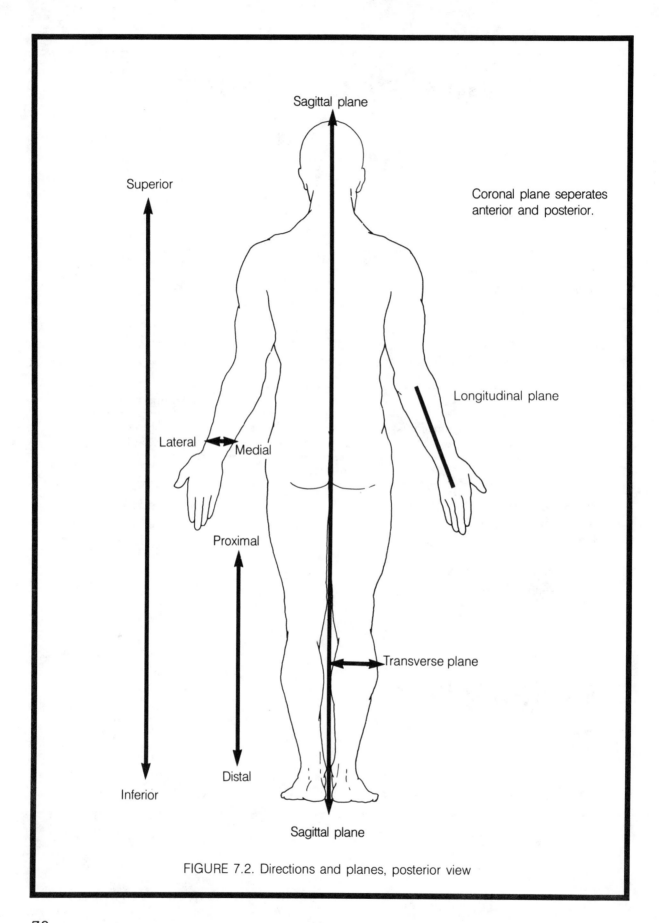

FIGURE 7.2. Directions and planes, posterior view

	Aids to Learning		
Term	**Anatomical Use**	**Illustrative Words**	**Literal Meaning**
Directions			
cephalic, superior (se-FAL-ik)	above		cephal = head
caudal, inferior (KAW-dal)	below		caud = tail
internal	inside		
external	outside		
intrinsic (in-TRIN-sik)	belonging entirely to one structure		
extrinsic (eks-TRIN-sik)	on outside of a structure in the body		
superficial (soo-per-FISH-al)	toward the surface		
deep	away from the surface		
dextral (DEKS-tral)	right	dexterity	
sinistral (SIN-is-tral)	left	sinister	
Planes			
sagittal (SAJ-i-tal)	dividing right and left	Sagittarius (Zodiac)	arrow
coronal, frontal (kō-RŌ-nal)	dividing anterior and posterior	coronation	coron = crown
transverse (trans-VERS)	dividing superior and inferior		turn across
longitudinal (lon-ji-TŪ-di-nal)	lengthwise		

TEST YOUR KNOWLEDGE

Section A

Define and give a synonym for each of the following.

		Definition	Synonym
1.	Cephalic	Above	superior
2.	Frontal	~ing Anterior & posterior	coronal
3.	Posterior	back	dorsal
4.	Ventral	front	Anterior
5.	Inferior	below	Caudal

Section B

Give terms used for the following definitions.

1. Dividing superior and inferior — transverse
2. Toward the surface — superficial
3. Near to — proximal
4. Dividing right and left — sagittal
5. Side — lateral
6. Inside — internal
7. Dividing anterior and posterior — frontal & coronal
8. Lengthwise — longitudinal
9. Far from — distal
10. Middle — mesial & medial

Section C

Write the proper term in the blank to indicate the spatial relationship of body parts in anatomical position (standing with palms to the front).

1. The head is the ____(cephalic) superior____ end of the body.
2. The waist is ____(caudal) inferior____ to the neck.
3. A ____transverse____ plane would separate the head from the body.
4. The cheeks are ____lateral____ to the nose.
5. The skin is ____superficial____ to the muscles.
6. The wrist is ____distal____ (proximal or distal) to the elbow.
7. The breastbone is ____medial____ to the nipples.
8. The navel is on the ____ventral____ surface of the body.
9. The leg is ____proximal____ (proximal or distal) to the foot.

40

10. A _____coronal (frontal)_____ plane would separate the face from the rest of the head.

11. The buttocks are on the _____posterior_____ side of the body.

12. The sole of the foot is on the _____(caudal) inferior_____ end of the body.

13. A _____transverse_____ plane through the arm would divide the hand from the shoulder.

14. The hips are in a _____medial lateral_____ position in the body.

15. A _____Sagittal_____ plane would divide the body into right and left halves.

Answers to Lesson 7—page 216

On the following pages are diagrams of directions and planes for you to label.

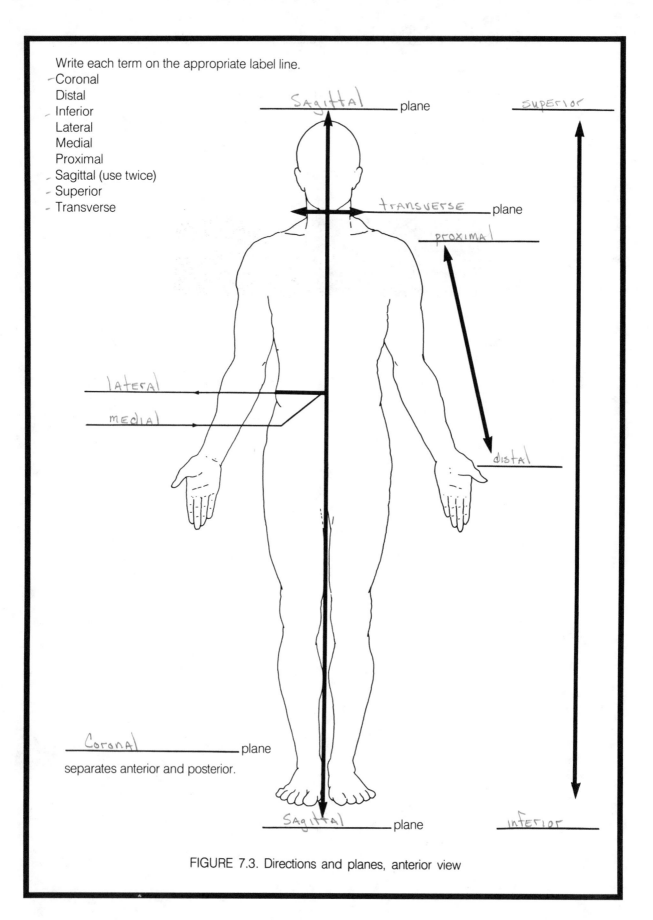

Write each term on the appropriate label line.
- Coronal
- Distal
- Inferior
- Lateral
- Medial
- Proximal
- Sagittal (use twice)
- Superior
- Transverse

Sagittal _____ plane

Superior _____

transverse _____ plane

Proximal _____

lateral _____

medial _____

distal _____

Coronal _____ plane
separates anterior and posterior.

Sagittal _____ plane

inferior _____

FIGURE 7.3. Directions and planes, anterior view

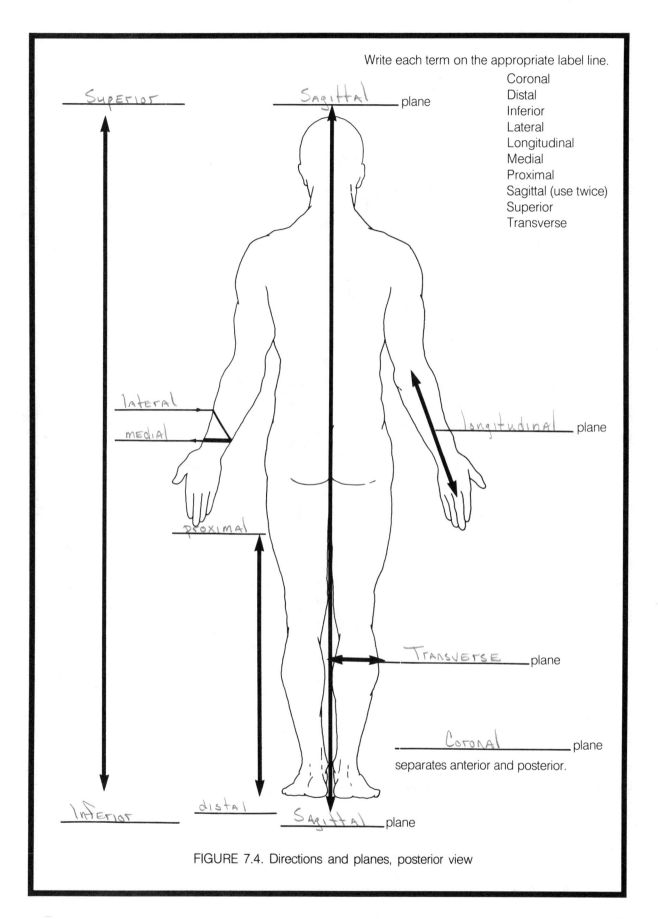

Write each term on the appropriate label line.

Coronal
Distal
Inferior
Lateral
Longitudinal
Medial
Proximal
Sagittal (use twice)
Superior
Transverse

Superior

Sagittal plane

lateral

medial

proximal

longitudinal plane

Transverse plane

Coronal plane separates anterior and posterior.

Inferior

distal

Sagittal plane

FIGURE 7.4. Directions and planes, posterior view

43

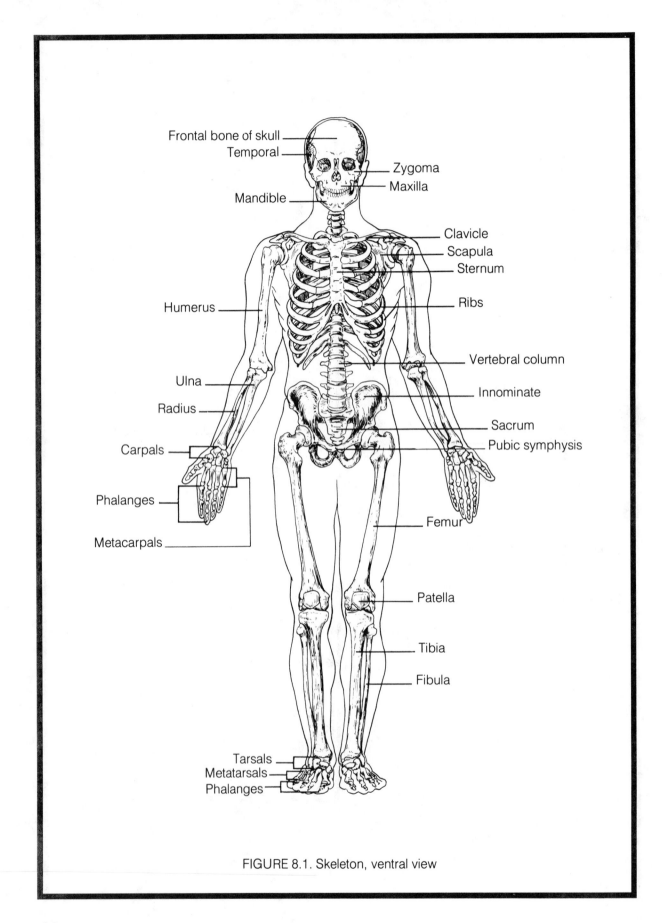

Frontal bone of skull

Temporal

Zygoma

Maxilla

Mandible

Clavicle

Scapula

Sternum

Humerus

Ribs

Vertebral column

Ulna

Radius

Innominate

Sacrum

Pubic symphysis

Carpals

Phalanges

Metacarpals

Femur

Patella

Tibia

Fibula

Tarsals

Metatarsals

Phalanges

FIGURE 8.1. Skeleton, ventral view

Skeleton and Muscle

Skeleton: from Greek, meaning dried up body
Muscle: from Latin, meaning little mouse

The skeletal system is the basic structural framework of the body. Its 206 *bones*, together with the *ligaments* that bind them together, perform such functions as supporting soft tissues and protecting internal organs. They also provide a firm base for attachment of muscles so that muscle contraction effects movement. In addition, the red marrow, a soft tissue within certain bones, manufactures a number of different kinds of blood cells, and bones act as storage areas for mineral salts and fat.

The skeleton is divided into *axial* and *appendicular* portions. The major parts of the axial skeleton are the *skull, vertebral column, ribs,* and *sternum* (i.e., the bones of the head, neck, and trunk). The bones in the appendages and those in the trunk that support them make up the appendicular skeleton.

Junctions between bones, called *joints* or *articulations*, are variously structured; some are rigid, such as most of those in the skull, but most afford various degrees of motion, ranging up to such freely movable areas as the shoulder and hip. *Cartilage* is associated with many joints and is thus considered with the skeletal system.

The muscular system is composed of those muscles that are called *skeletal* because they have one or more attachments to bones, usually by means of *tendons*. When a muscle contracts it shortens and, since the tendon does not stretch, a bone is moved. The approximately 700 muscles are of many different shapes and sizes. They produce motions described by such terms as flexion and extension, abduction and adduction, elevation and depression, and rotation. The names of muscles may reflect these actions, or they may reflect such characteristics as the number and place of their attachments or the direction in which they run. A muscle usually performs its function not in isolation but as part of a group. In most parts of the body there are groups that oppose one another in their action. This antagonism allows for smoothness of motion and is coordinated by the nervous system.

		Aids to Learning	
Combining Form	**Anatomical Use**	**Common Name**	**Literal Meaning**
		General	
osteo- (OS-tē-ō)	bone		
chondro- (KON-drō)	cartilage	gristle	
arthro-, articulo- (AR-thrō) (ar-TIK-ū-lō)	joint		

45

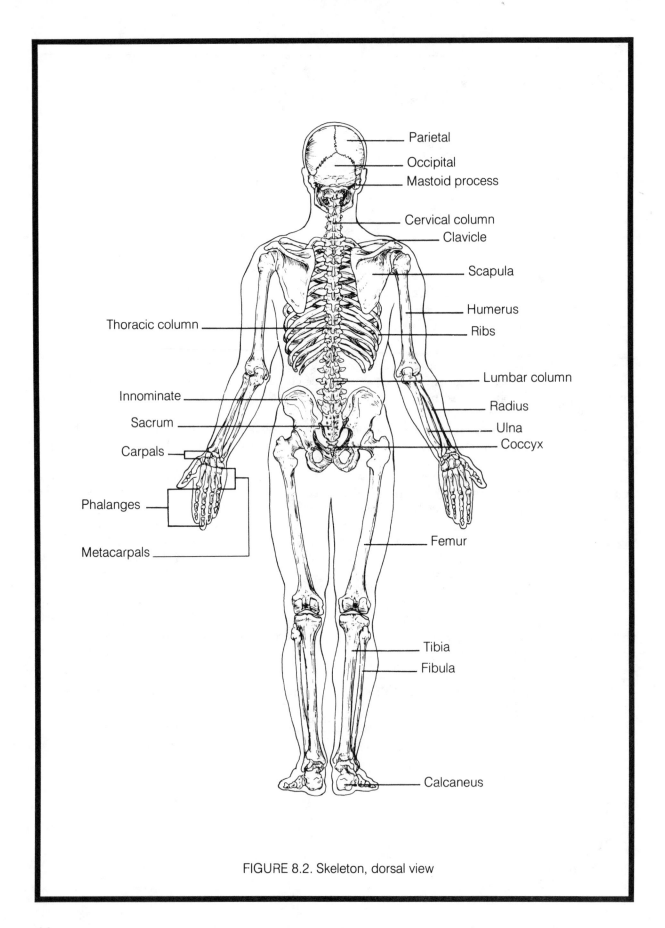

Parietal

Occipital

Mastoid process

Cervical column

Clavicle

Scapula

Humerus

Ribs

Thoracic column

Lumbar column

Innominate

Radius

Sacrum

Ulna

Coccyx

Carpals

Phalanges

Metacarpals

Femur

Tibia

Fibula

Calcaneus

FIGURE 8.2. Skeleton, dorsal view

	Aids to Learning		
Combining Form	**Anatomical Use**	**Common Name**	**Literal Meaning**

General

synovio- (si-NŌ-vē-ō)	joint fluid		with egg (fluid resembles egg white)
myelo-, medullo- (MĪ-e-lō) (me-DUL-ō)	marrow		
teno-, tendino- (TEN-ō) (TEN-di-nō)	tendon	sinew	
syndesmo- (sin-DES-mō)	ligament		bind with
sarco-	skeletal muscle	flesh	
myo- (MĪ-ō)	muscle		
fascio- (FASH-ē-ō)	fascia	muscle covering	band, bandage

Selected Skeletal Parts

cranio- (KRĀ-nē-ō)	cranium	skull	
rachi-, rachio-, spino- (RA-kē), (SPĪ-nō)	spinal column, vertebral column	backbone, spine	
spondylo- (SPON-di-lō)	vertebra		
sacro- (SĀ-krō)	sacrum		sacred
coccygo- (KOK-sē-gō)	coccyx	tailbone	cuckoo (resembles bill)
scapulo- (SKAP-ū-lō)	scapula	shoulder blade	
cleido-, clavico- (KLĪ-dō) (KLAV-i-kō)	clavicle	collarbone	cleid = hook clavic = key

	Aids to Learning		
Combining Form	Anatomical Use	Common Name	Literal Meaning
Selected Skeletal Parts			
sterno- (STER-nō)	sternum	breastbone	chest
costo- (KOS-tō)	rib		
humero- (HŪ-mer-ō)	humerus	armbone	upper arm
radio- (RĀ-dē-ō)	radius	forearm bone	ray
ulno- (UL-nō)	ulna	forearm bone	elbow
carpo- (KAR-pō)	carpus	wrist bones	
metacarpo- (me-ta-KAR-pō)	metacarpus	hand bones	after the wrist
femoro- (FEM-ō-rō)	femur	thighbone	thigh
patello- (pa-TEL-ō)	patella	kneecap	little dish
tibio- (TI-bē-ō)	tibia	shinbone	flute
peroneo-, fibulo- (per-ō-NĒ-ō) (FIB-ū-lō)	fibula		clasp, buckle, pin
tarso- (TAR-sō)	tarsus	ankle bones	broad, flat surface
metatarso- (me-ta-TAR-sō)	metatarsus	foot bones	after the ankle
phalango- (fa-LAN-gō)	phalanges	bones of fingers and toes	closely knit row

		Aids to Learning	
Combining Form	**Anatomical Use**	**Common Name**	**Literal Meaning**
Innominate Bone (Pelvic Bone) Parts			
ilio- (IL-ē-ō)	ilium	hipbone	groin, flank
ischio- (IS-kē-ō)	ischium		hip
pubo- (PŪ-bō)	pubis		grownup
pelvi-, pelvo-	pelvis (innominates and sacrum)		basin

WORDS USING THESE ELEMENTS

Record words given in class or encountered in your reading.

Word	**Meaning**
_____	_____
_____	_____
_____	_____
_____	_____
_____	_____
_____	_____
_____	_____
_____	_____
_____	_____
_____	_____

TEST YOUR KNOWLEDGE

Section A

Give the combining form for the following bones, given here by common name.

1. Thigh bone _____femoral_____
2. Hip bone _____
3. Skull _____
4. Collar bone _____clavico_____
5. Bones of fingers and toes _____phlango_____
6. Rib _____costo_____
7. Wrist bones _____carpo_____
8. Spinal column _____
9. Breastbone _____sterno_____
10. Shoulder blade _____scapulo_____
11. Hand bones _____metacarpo_____
12. Arm bone _____
13. Ankle bones _____tarso_____
14. Shin bone _____
15. Kneecap _____

Section B

Divide and define the following terms.

1. Polymyositis _____inflammation of many muscles_____
2. Medullary _____pertaining to the ~~medulla~~ MARROW_____
3. Intracranial _____within the cranium_____
4. Spondylosis _____(abnormal) condition of the vertebra_____
5. Chondroblast _____breaking down cartilage_____
6. Pelvimetry _____measurement of the pelvis_____
7. Synovial _____pertaining to joint fluid_____
8. Disarticular _____pertaining to ~~bad painful~~ joints_____
9. Periosteum _____
10. Subscapular _____pertaining to below the scapula_____
11. Coccygeal _____pertaining to coccyx_____
12. Syndesmosis _____
13. Osteolysis _____destruction of bone_____

50

14. Rachianesthesia _without physical sensation in the vertebra_ *vert*

15. Fasciectomy _removal of_

16. Peroneal _pertaining to_

17. Pubic symphysis _pubis grow together_
(sym- is a softened form of syn- used before b, m, and p)

18. Intercostal _between the ribs_

19. Myelogenesis _formation of ~~muscle~~ MARROW_

20. Arthritis _inflammation of the joints_

21. Osteomyelitis _inflammation of bone MARROW ~~and muscle~~_

22. Substernal _pertaining to below the sternum_

Section C

Complete the following terms.

1. Extra_____ _crani_ _____ al   outside the skull

2. _____ _peri_ ___synovitis   inflammation of the membrane around a tendon

3. _____ pexy   fixation of a ligament

4. _____ _sarco_ ___ lemma   covering of skeletal muscle (fiber)

5. Peri _____ _chondr_ ___ ium   (membrane) around cartilage

6. _____ phrenic   pertaining to ribs and diaphragm

7. _____al   pertaining to bones of wrist and hand

8. _____ form   shaped like the kneecap

9. _____ ar joint   joint between the bones of the forearm

10. _____ oma   tumor of bone marrow

11. _____ asthenic   pertaining to muscle weakness

12. _____ odynia   pain in the spine

13. _____ malacia   softening of a vertebra

Answers to Lesson 8—page 217

On the following pages are:

1. Two views of the skeleton. On each label line, write in the name of the bone.

2. Two views of the body indicating the names of many muscles. Practice using your terminology by seeing how many muscle names you can analyze.

Write each combining form on the appropriate label line.

Carpo-
Cleido-, claviculo-
Costo-
Cranio-
Femoro-
Humero-
Ilio-
Ischio-
Metacarpo-
Metatarso-
Patello-

Peroneo-, fibulo-
Pelvi-, pelvo-
Phalango- (use twice)
Pubo-
Radio-
Sacro-
Sterno-
Tarso-
Tibio-
Ulno-

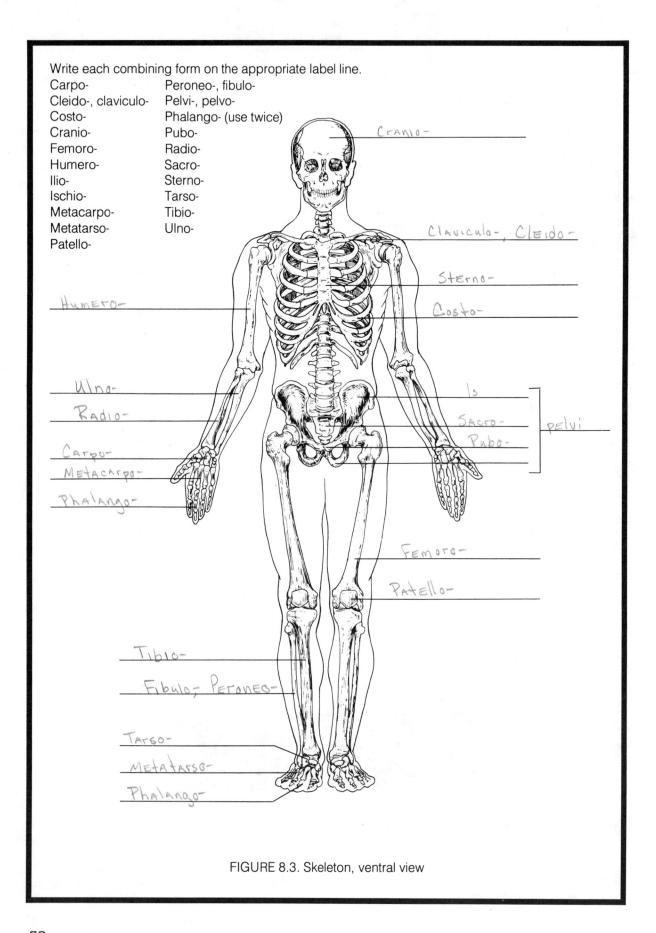

Cranio-
Claviculo-, Cleido-
Sterno-
Costo-
Humero-
Ulno-
Radio-
Carpo-
Metacarpo-
Phalango-
Is
Sacro-
Pubo-
Pelvi
Femoro-
Patello-
Tibio-
Fibulo-, Peroneo-
Tarso-
Metatarso-
Phalango-

FIGURE 8.3. Skeleton, ventral view

52

Write each combining form on the appropriate label line.

Carpo- Peroneo-, fibulo-
Cleido-, claviculo- Phalango-
Coccygo- Rachi-, spino-
Costo- Radio-
Cranio- Sacro-
Femoro- Scapulo-
Humero- Tarso-
Ilio- Tibio-
Ischio- Ulno-
Metacarpo-

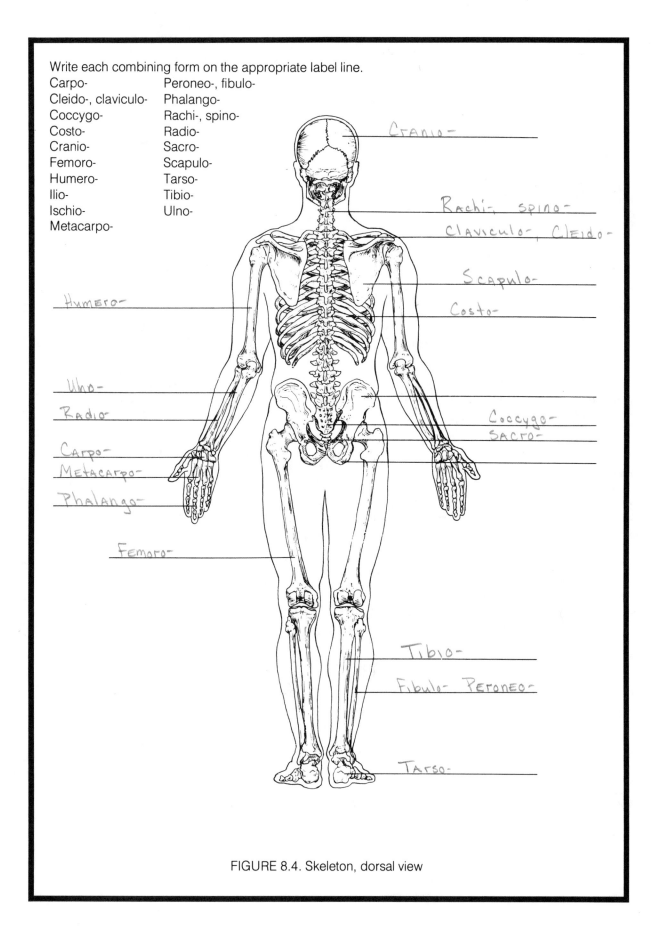

Cranio-

Rachi-, spino-
Claviculo-, Cleido-

Scapulo-

Costo-

Humero-

Ulno-

Radio-

Coccygo-
Sacro-

Carpo-
Metacarpo-
Phalango-

Femoro-

Tibio-

Fibulo- Peroneo-

Tarso-

FIGURE 8.4. Skeleton, dorsal view

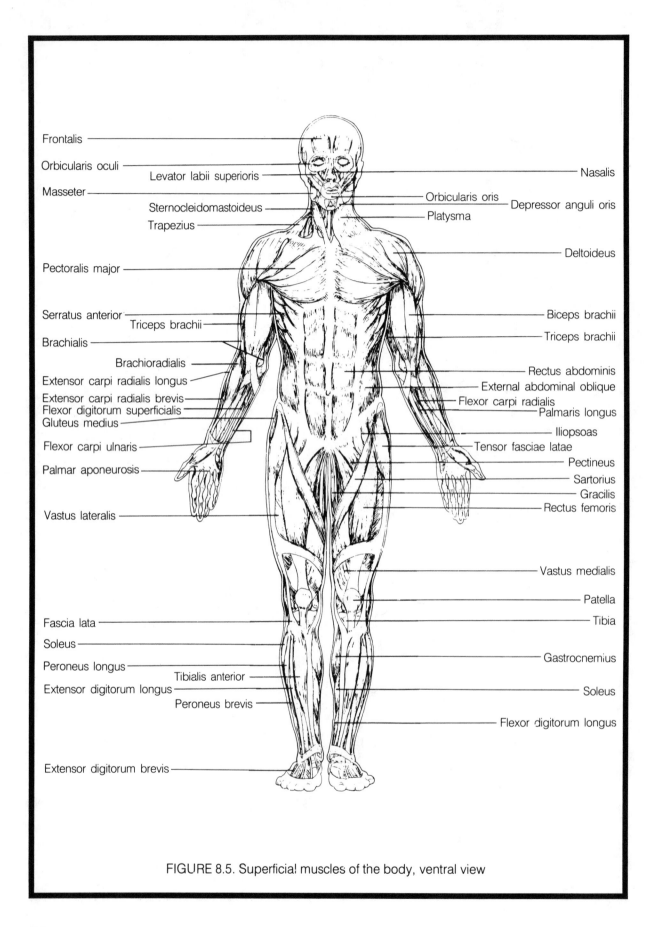

Frontalis

Orbicularis oculi

Levator labii superioris

Masseter

Sternocleidomastoideus

Trapezius

Pectoralis major

Serratus anterior

Triceps brachii

Brachialis

Brachioradialis

Extensor carpi radialis longus

Extensor carpi radialis brevis

Flexor digitorum superficialis

Gluteus medius

Flexor carpi ulnaris

Palmar aponeurosis

Vastus lateralis

Fascia lata

Soleus

Peroneus longus

Extensor digitorum longus

Tibialis anterior

Peroneus brevis

Extensor digitorum brevis

Nasalis

Orbicularis oris

Depressor anguli oris

Platysma

Deltoideus

Biceps brachii

Triceps brachii

Rectus abdominis

External abdominal oblique

Flexor carpi radialis

Palmaris longus

Iliopsoas

Tensor fasciae latae

Pectineus

Sartorius

Gracilis

Rectus femoris

Vastus medialis

Patella

Tibia

Gastrocnemius

Soleus

Flexor digitorum longus

FIGURE 8.5. Superficial muscles of the body, ventral view

54

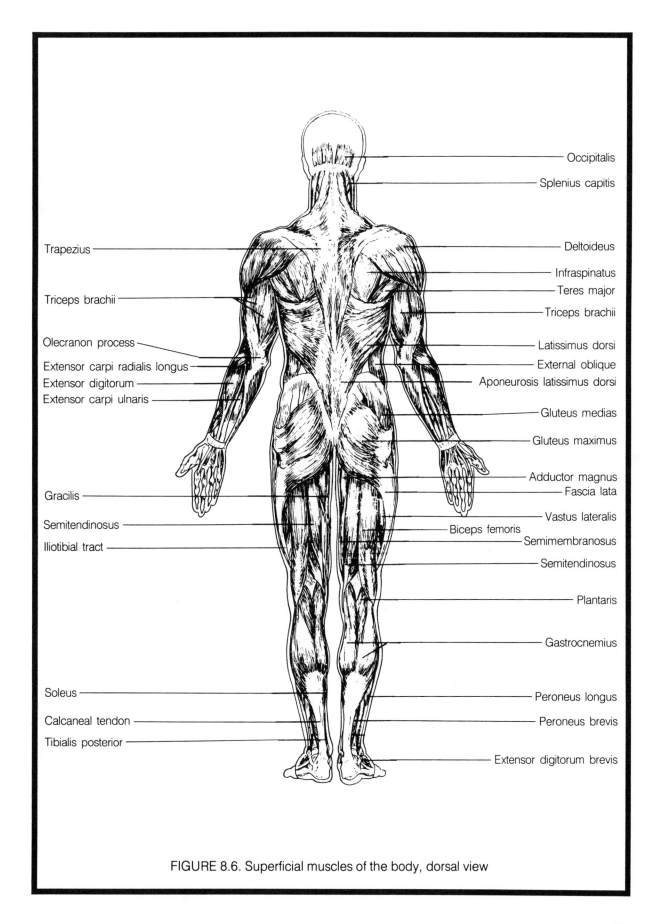

Occipitalis

Splenius capitis

Trapezius

Deltoideus

Infraspinatus

Teres major

Triceps brachii

Triceps brachii

Olecranon process

Latissimus dorsi

Extensor carpi radialis longus

External oblique

Extensor digitorum

Aponeurosis latissimus dorsi

Extensor carpi ulnaris

Gluteus medias

Gluteus maximus

Gracilis

Adductor magnus

Fascia lata

Semitendinosus

Vastus lateralis

Iliotibial tract

Biceps femoris

Semimembranosus

Semitendinosus

Plantaris

Gastrocnemius

Soleus

Peroneus longus

Calcaneal tendon

Peroneus brevis

Tibialis posterior

Extensor digitorum brevis

FIGURE 8.6. Superficial muscles of the body, dorsal view

55

Pathologies

Patho: from Greek, meaning disease	

Listing all disease conditions here would be impossible. What follows is just a selection of those most frequently encountered. Note that some elements listed are used as prefixes, some are used as suffixes, and a few are used as separate words.

		Aids to Learning
Word Element	**Meaning**	**Illustrative Words**
-algia, -odynia (AL-jē-a) (ō-DIN-ē-a)	pain	neuralgia
-algesia (al-JĒ-zē-a)	sensation of pain	analgesic
ankylo- (ANG-ki-lō)	stiffness	
-asthenia (as-THĒ-nē-a)	weakness	myasthenia gravis
brady- (BRAD-ē)	slow	
carcino- (KAR-si-nō)	cancer	carcinogenic
-cele (sēl)	herniation	
-ectasia, -ectasis (ek-TĀ-zē-a) (EK-ta-sis)	dilatation	
-ectopia, -ectopy (ek-TŌ-pē-a) (EK-tō-pē)	displacement	ectopic pregnancy
edema (e-DĒ-ma)	swelling	edematous

Word Element	Meaning	Aids to Learning Illustrative Words
-emia (Ē-mē-a)	condition of blood	toxemia, septicemia
-itis (Ī-tis)	inflammation	arthritis
-lepsy (LEP-sē)	seizure	epilepsy
-lith, litho-, calculo- (LITH-ō) (KAL-kū-lō)	stone	lithographer, renal calculus
-lysis (LĪ-sis)	destruction	hemolysis
-malacia (ma-LĀ-shē-ā)	softening	
mania (MĀ-nē-a)	obsessive preoccupation	megalomania
-megaly (ME-ga-lē)	enlargement	
narco- (NAR-kō)	numbness	narcotic
-oma, onco- (Ō-ma) (ON-kō)	tumor	carcinoma, oncology
-osis (Ō-sis)	condition (often abnormal)	
patho-, -pathy, morb- (PATH-ō)	disease	pathogenic, homeopathy, morbidity
-penia (PĒ-nē-a)	deficiency	
-phobia (FŌ-bē-a)	fear	hydrophobia

	Aids to Learning	
Word Element	Meaning	Illustrative Words
-plegia (PLE-jē-a)	paralysis	hemiplegia
-ptosis (TŌ-sis)	drooping	
pyro-, pyreto- febri- (PĪ-rō) (pī-RE-tō) (FEB-ri)	fever	antipyretic
-rrhagia (RĀ-jē-a)	extreme flow	hemorrhage
-rrhexis (REK-sis)	rupture	
schizo-, -schisis (SKIZ-ō) (SKI-sis)	splitting	schizophrenia
-sclerosis (skle-RŌ-sis)	hardening	arteriosclerosis
-sepsis (SEP-sis)	infection	asepsis, antiseptic
-spasm	spasm	
-stenosis (ste-NŌ-sis)	stricture	
tachy- (TAK-ē)	fast	tachycardia
-uria (Ū-rē-a)	condition of urine	hematuria

WORDS USING THESE ELEMENTS

Record words given in class or encountered in your reading.

Word	Meaning

TEST YOUR KNOWLEDGE

Section A

Select from the list the pathological condition that is indicated by each word element and write it in the blank.

1. -lepsy _____ SEIZURE _____   tumor
2. -cele _____ herniation _____   fear
3. -sepsis _____ infection _____   weakness
4. -odynia _____ pain _____   dilatation
5. -phobia _____ fear _____   stone
6. Pyro- _____ fever _____   stricture
7. -rrhagia _____ Extreme flow _____   fast
8. -asthenia _____ weakness _____   seizure
9. -lith _____ stone _____   stiffness
10. Onco- _____ tumor _____   deficiency
11. Tachy- _____ Fast _____   extreme flow
12. Ankylo- _____ stiffness _____   fever

60

13. -penia ___deficiency___   infection

14. -ectasia ___dilatation___   pain

15. -stenosis ___stricture___   herniation

Section B

Divide and define the following.

1. Narcolepsy ___numbing seizure___
2. Analgesia ___without sensation of pain___
3. Ankyloarthrosis ___condition of stiffness in joints___
4. Myorrhexis ___muscle rupture___
5. Pathogenic ___disease producing (forming)___
6. Pyrophobia ___fear of fever___
7. Hemiplegia ___half (partial) paralysis___
8. Visceroptosis ___drooping viscera (internal organs)___
9. Osteomalacia ___bone softening___
10. Spondylitis ___inflammation of VERTEBRA___
11. Cranioschisis ___cranial splitting___
12. Antisepsis ___against infection___
13. Myospasm ___muscle spasm___
14. Menorrhagia ___extreme menstrual flow___
15. Cephalomegaly ___enlargement of head___

Section C

Complete the following definitions.

1. Orchid/ectopy ___displacement___ of the testis
2. Tox/emia poison in the ___blood___
3. Renal calculus kidney ___stone___
4. Esophag/o/stenosis ___narrowing dilatation___ of the esophagus
5. Hemat/uria blood in the ___urine___
6. Chole/cyst/algia ___pain___ in the gall bladder
7. Path/o/genic producing ___disease___
8. Neur/asthenia nerve ___weakness___
9. Brady/lexia ___slow___ reading
10. Febrile characterized by ___fever___

61

Section D

Complete the following terms.

1. Pyro _MANIA_ — obsessive occupation with fire

2. _Trachy_ cardia — fast heart

3. Blepharo _ptosis_ — drooping of the eyelid

4. Arterio _sclerosis_ — hardening of the arteries

5. Myx _edemia_ — mucous swelling

6. Phlebo _rrhexis_ — rupture of a vein

7. Carcino _phobia_ — fear of cancer

8. Cysto _cele_ — herniation of the bladder

9. Leuko _penia_ — deficiency of white (cells)

10. _Anklylo_ glossia — stiffness of tongue

Answers to Lesson 9—page 218

TERMINOLOGY SEARCH 1: A MEDICAL PAPER

Continuous research efforts underlie modern medicine; results of such research are published in medical journals. This example is from *Virginia Medical*.

Osteogenic Sarcoma Occurring after Irradiation

Richard H. Fitzgerald, Jr., MD, *Charleston, South Carolina,*
and Tapan A. Hazra, MD, *Richmond*

IONIZING irradiation can produce necrosis, growth arrest, fracture, and benign as well as malignant neoplasm in bone.[1] The most common osseous malignant tumor to develop in the irradiated area is osteosarcoma, although fibrosarcoma and chondrosarcoma do occur.[2] Reported here is the case history of a patient who received irradiation as a child and 13 years later experienced several long-term sequelae, including osteosarcoma.

Case Report

In December 1966 a 12-month-old boy developed a nodule in the posterior lumbar paraspinal musculature. At age 15 months he underwent excision of a 2.5-cm embryonal rhabdomyosarcoma, with 5-10 mitotic figures per high-powered microscopic field. At age 19 months multiple small nodules appeared in the area of surgical scar, and he received 5987 rad tumor dose (TD) in 41 treatments over 61 days by shrinking fields to the left of the midline from L2 to L5 with two MeV photons; to achieve the most effective treatment, all the irradiation was delivered from

This article was begun when Dr. Fitzgerald was a fellow at the Medical College of Virginia under the direction of Dr. Hazra, chairman of the Division of Radiation Therapy and Oncology. Dr. Fitzgerald is now with the Medical University of South Carolina and may be addressed there at the Division of Radiation Therapy, 171 Ashley Avenue, Charleston, SC 29403.

Supported in part by the American Cancer Society, Clinical Fellow #3232A and Grant #5R-25CA22032-02 awarded by the National Cancer Institute.

Submitted 7-14-80.

the back of the patient. Following this, chemotherapy of actinomycin D, vincristine and cyclophosphamide was begun and continued until local recurrence was noted in June 1968, 15 months after excision and 9 months after completion of irradiation. Wide surgical excision of the area was performed. No other therapy was given, and the patient was subsequently lost to followup.

Seen for an unrelated problem in January 1979 at age 12, the patient was found to have an asymptomatic mass in the left lower quadrant contiguous with the left iliac bone. Roentgenographs demonstrated the left ilium to be smaller than the right and to contain an osteoblastic lesion (Fig. 1). There was scoliosis toward the side of prior irradiation. Intravenous pylogram demonstrated atrophy of the lower one-half of the left kidney and hypertrophy of the right kidney (Fig. 2). Chest tomography and CT scan were normal. Alkaline phosphatase was normal for age 12 at 180, SGOT was 79, and LDH 379. In late January 1979, he underwent left hemi-pelvectomy after biopsy confirmation of sarcoma. There was a 7×9×6-cm mass of chondroblastic osteosarcoma superficially invading the muscle in the area of biopsy. Ten days following surgery, he was begun on adjuvant doxorubicin hydrochloride (Adriamycin®). In mid-1980, more than one year after surgery and chemotherapy, there was no evidence of recurrence or metastasis.

Discussion

Marie in 1910 described sarcomas in irradiated animals.[1] In 1922 Beck and Marsch independently re-

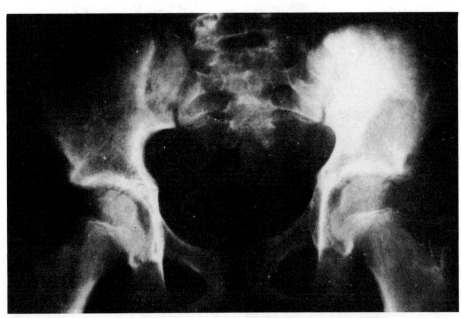

Fig. 1. Roentgenograph of 12-year-old patient shows osteosarcoma in hypoplastic left ilium.

ported bone sarcomas in humans treated for tuberculous arthritis.[2] Martland in 1929 reported two radium-dial painters who developed sarcoma.[3] A higher than expected rate of bone tumor was recorded by Court-Brown and Doll[4] in 1965 in patients treated with external irradiation for ankylosing spondylitis; they questioned, however, the validity of this increase because of the dependence on death certificate statements.

In 1948 Cahan[5] described cases of irradiation-related bone sarcoma with four criteria in common:

1) Microscopic or radiographic evidence of the initial non-malignant nature of the involved bone.
2) Sarcomas developed in areas previously included within radiotherapeutic beams.
3) All sarcomas were proven histologically.
4) A relatively long asymptomatic latent period (greater than five years) elapsed after irradiation before the clinical appearance of the sarcoma.

Modifications of Cahan's criteria have been proposed. Senyszyn[6] suggested that roentgenographic evidence of osteodysplasia more than one year prior to the onset of obvious malignancy would not be seen with spontaneous neoplasm and implied that prior x-ray studies were required for positive implication of

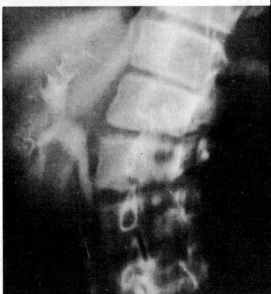

Fig. 2. Intravenous pyelogram of same patient, showing hypoplastic left kidney and scoliosis.

Table 1. Occurrence of Osteogenic Sarcoma in Irradiated Survivors of Prior Malignancy.

Group	Number at Risk	occurrence	Occurrence Rate
General Population[11,13]	117,000	1	0.00085%
Sagerman[10]			
Retinoblastoma	243	9	3.7%
Tountas[9]	29,000	10	0.035%
Cervix	3,500	2	0.06%
Breast	8,000	4	0.05%
Hatfield, Schulz[11]			
Breast	900	2	0.22%
	(estimate)		
Phillips, Sheline[12]	2,300	2	0.1%
Cervix	505	1	0.2%
Breast	445	1	0.22%

irradiation. Cohen[7] described a juxtacortical lucency in a rib two years after therapy for Wilm's tumor, with a sarcoma diagnosed one year later, or three years after therapy. Arlen[1] also described cases with a shorter latent period and included reticulum cell and Ewing's sarcomas, thus expanding Cahan's criteria to include sarcomas devoid of osteoblastic activity. Doses as low as 1200 rad have been incriminated, though most have followed greater than 3000 rad.

The neoplastic hazard following irradiation of a large portion of the skeleton appears to be leukemia or a related hematological disorder, but for limited field exposure a bone malignancy is more likely. The area of endosteal surface is much greater than the area of periosteal surface, and when studied, osteogenic sarcoma does appear to arise from the endosteal surface.[2] A hypocellular marrow with hyperplastic fibroblasts interspersed with practically intact bone suggests that the sarcomatous change occurs in areas of intermediate damage.[8] All bones of the skeleton are at risk.[1,7,9]

Continued long-term followup of large registries of patients is needed to provide meaningful occurrence rates for osteogenic sarcoma. The available data of 3- to 10-year followup are helpful, however, and incidence seems to increase with dose.[9,10]

Tountas[9] concluded the incidence to be 0.05-0.2% among survivors given current therapeutic dosages of 4000-7000 rad. He reported ten cases among 29,000 5-year survivors, providing a crude rate of 1 in 2900 (0.035%) for all patients; included were two women among 3500 5-year survivors of breast cancer therapy (0.05%). Hatfield and Schulz[11] reported an incidence of 0.22% among their 10-year survivors of breast cancer treatment. Phillips and Sheline[12] saw an incidence of 0.1% in 2300 5-year survivors.

To place these figures in perspective, the spontaneous rate is one case in 117,000[13] to one in 200,000[11] in the general population. These figures indicate a 41- to 258-fold increase in occurrence rate in irradiated patients compared with the general population, a significant finding at the $P < .01$ level (Table 1). Sagerman et al[10] reported nine cases of osteogenic sarcoma among 243 patients irradiated for retinoblastoma; this incidence (3.7%) reflects the apparent increased susceptibility of patients with retinoblastoma to osteosarcoma both within and removed from the irradiated site.[11,13] After irradiation, patients apparently cured of localized Ewing's sarcoma have an increased incidence of osteogenic sarcoma in the treated bone.[14]

Radical surgery is the preferred treatment for radiation-induced osteosarcoma,[1] but when surgery has not been possible, radiation has been used with transient palliative benefit.[1,8]

No series has addressed the role of chemotherapy in radiation-induced osteogenic sarcoma; in one case where it was used, there was transient and partial pain relief.[15]

The prognosis of radiation-induced lesions appears to parallel that of spontaneous osteogenic sarcoma. Dahlin[16] reported a survival rate of 20.3% of his total series and 17.3% of patients with radiation-induced lesions. Arlen[1] reported a survival rate of 17.8% of all cases (552) and 28% (14 of 50) of patients with radiation-related disease.

The authors gratefully acknowledge the assistance of Dr. C. Russell and Dr. J. Terz, who supplied followup data, and C. B. Loadholt, who provided statistical assistance.

References

1. Arlen M, Higinbotham NL, Huvos AG et al: Radiation induced sarcoma of bone. Cancer: 1087-1099, 1971
2. Vaughan JM: The Effects of Irradiation on the Skeleton. Oxford, Clarendon Press, 1973
3. Martland HS, Humphries RE: Osteogenic sarcoma in dial painters using luminous paint. Arch Pathol 7:406-417, 1929
4. Court-Brown WM, Doll R: Mortality from cancer and other causes after radiotherapy for ankylosing spondylitis. Brit Med J 2:1327-1332, 1965
5. Cahan WG, Woodard HQ, Higinbotham ND et al: Sarcoma arising in bone: report of eleven cases. Cancer 1: 3-29, 1948
6. Senyszyn JJ, Johnston AD, Jacox HW et al: Radiation induced sarcoma after treatment of breast carcinoma. Cancer 26: 394-403, 1970
7. Cohen J, D'Angio GJ: Bone tumors after roentgen therapy. Am J Radiol 86:502-512, 1961
8. Cruz M, Coley BL, Stewart FW: Post radiation bone sarcoma: report of eleven cases. Cancer 10: 72-87, 1957
9. Tountas AA, Fornasier VL, Harwood AR et al: Post irradiation sarcoma of bone: a perspective. Cancer 43:182-187, 1979
10. Sagerman RH, Cassady JR, Tretter P et al: Radiation

induced neoplasia following external beam therapy for children with retinoblastoma. Amer J Radiol 105:529-535, 1969

11. Hatfield PM, Schulz MD: Post irradiation sarcoma. Radiol 96: 593-602, 1970

12. Phillips TL, Sheline GE: Bone sarcomas following radiation therapy. Radiol 81: 992-996, 1963

13. Abramson DH, Ellsworth RM, Zimmerman LE: Non-ocular cancer in retinoblastoma survivors. Proc Am Acad Ophthalmol Otolaryngol 81:454-457, 1976

14. Chan RC, Sutow WW, Lindberg RD et al: Management and results of localized Ewing's sarcoma. Cancer 43:1001-1006, 1979

15. Tewfik H, Tewfik F, Latourette H et al: Radiotherapy induced rib osteosarcoma after successful treatment of lung cancer. Radiol 125:503-504, 1977

16. Dahlin DC: Bone Tumors, 2nd Ed. Springfield, Illinois, Charles C. Thomas, 1967, pp 156-176

From *Virginia Medical*, vol. 108, pp. 474-477. Reprinted by permission of the authors and publisher.

Nervous System

Nerve: from Latin, meaning sinew (tendon, similar to nerve in appearance)

In any complex organism such as the human body there must be some coordination of the large number of activities that take place at any given time. The nervous and endocrine systems, which are responsible for this coordination, complement each other nicely. The endocrine glands secrete hormones which are carried by the blood into all body tissues and play a major role in maintaining the necessary chemical activities of cells. By means of nerve impulses, the nervous system regulates the activity of muscles and glands and thus of almost all the body systems. Information about changes in the internal and external environment is sent to the central nervous system (*brain* and *spinal cord*), where it is processed and from which directions are sent out to the muscles and glands. This sequence of nerve impulses to and away from the brain or cord is called a *reflex*. It can be diagrammed simply as:

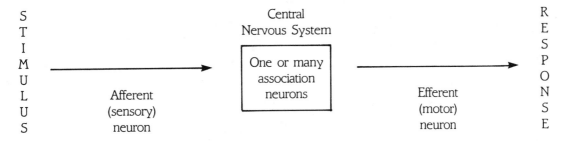

Together, the brain and spinal cord are called the central nervous system because they are central in location as well as function. They are protected by the skull and vertebral column, by membranes called *meninges*, and by *cerebrospinal fluid*. The central nervous system has internal cavities (called *ventricles* in the brain) that contain the same circulating fluid. Major brain parts are *cerebrum, cerebellum, thalamus, hypothalamus, midbrain, pons*, and *medulla*. The cranial nerves from the brain and the spinal nerves from the cord are collectively referred to as the *peripheral nervous system*, since they extend to all parts of the body. All parts of the nervous system contain *neurons*, the cells that carry the impulses.

The nerves that take directions to the glands and the muscles of the internal organs are called *autonomic*, since activity of these tissues usually is not under our control and therefore seems to be automatic. In contrast, the *somatic* nerves take impulses to the skeletal muscles, which are under our voluntary control.

Sense organs are those structures that can detect environmental change and start a nerve impulse. Some are microscopic neuron endings, but others such as the eye and ear are extremely complex, having structures that protect the neuron endings and insure that the stimulus reaches them in proper form.

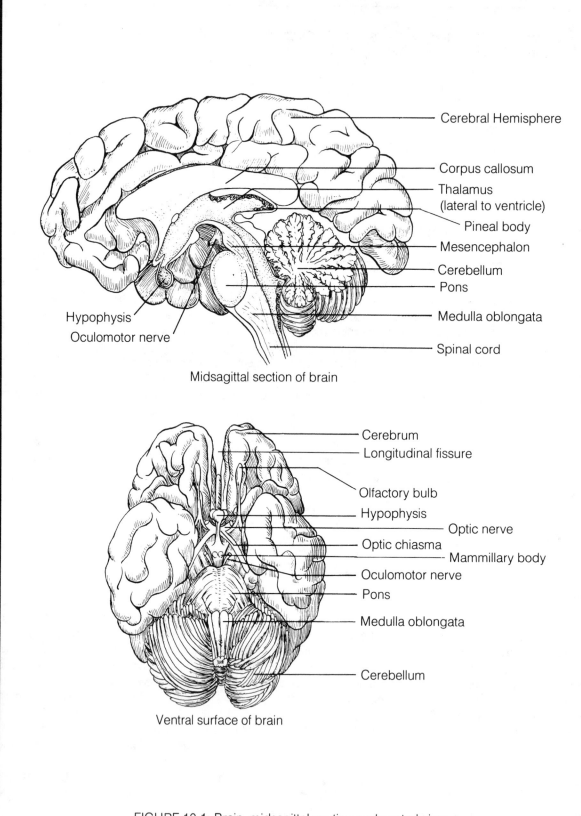

Cerebral Hemisphere

Corpus callosum

Thalamus
(lateral to ventricle)

Pineal body

Mesencephalon

Cerebellum

Pons

Medulla oblongata

Spinal cord

Hypophysis

Oculomotor nerve

Midsagittal section of brain

Cerebrum

Longitudinal fissure

Olfactory bulb

Hypophysis

Optic nerve

Optic chiasma

Mammillary body

Oculomotor nerve

Pons

Medulla oblongata

Cerebellum

Ventral surface of brain

FIGURE 10.1. Brain, midsagittal section and ventral view

	Aids to Learning		
Combining Form	Anatomical Use	Illustrative Words	Literal Meaning
neuro-, neuri (NŪ-rō)	nerve	neuralgia	sinew
ganglio- (GANG-glē-ō)	ganglion		swelling, knot
meningo- (me-NING-gō)	meninges	meningitis	membrane
encephalo- (en-SEF-a-lō)	brain	encephalitis	in head
cerebro- (SER-ē-brō)	cerebrum		brain
phreno-, psycho-, mento- (FRE-nō) (SĪ-kō) (MEN-tō)	mind	schizophrenia, psychology, mental	
cerebello- (ser-e-BEL-ō)	cerebellum		little brain
ponto- (PON-tō)	pons	pontoon	bridge
medullo- (me-DUL-ō)	medulla		marrow
ventriculo- (ven-TRIK-ū-lō)	ventricle		little belly
myelo-, spino- (MĪ-e-lō) (SPĪ-nō)	spinal cord	poliomyelitis, cerebrospinal	myelo = marrow
autonomo- (aw-tō-NOM-ō)	autonomic		self-law
tympano-, myringo- (TIM-pan-ō) (mi-RING-gō)	eardrum	timpani	drum
auriculo- (aw-RIK-ū-lō)	external ear		little ear
oto- (Ō-tō)	ear	otitis media	

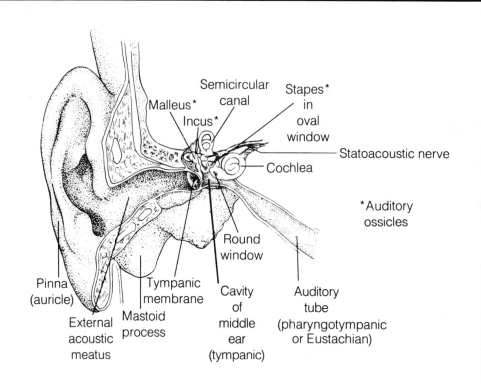

FIGURE 10.2. Inner ear, middle ear, and external ear

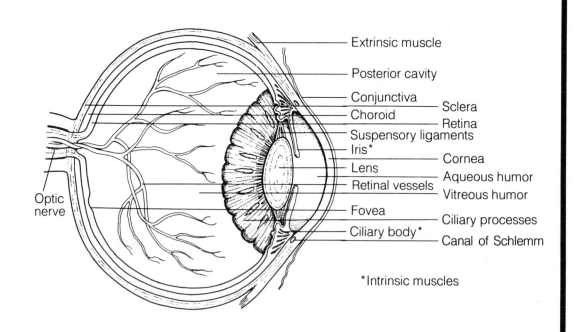

FIGURE 10.3. Eye, transverse section

Combining Form	Anatomical Use	Illustrative Words	Literal Meaning
cochleo- (KOK-lē-ō)	cochlea		snail
ophthalmo-, oculo- (of-THAL-mō) (OK-ū-lō)	eye	ophthalmology, oculist	
kerato-, corneo- (KER-a-tō) (KOR-nē-ō)	cornea	keratoplasty	horny
dacryo-, lacrimo- (DAK-rē-ō) (LAK-ri-mō)	tears	lacrimose	
retino- (RET-i-nō)	retina	retinopathy	network
conjunctivo- (kon-junk-TĪ-vō)	conjunctiva	conjunctivitis	join together

WORDS USING THESE ELEMENTS

Record words given in class or encountered in your reading.

Word	Meaning
_____	_____
_____	_____
_____	_____
_____	_____
_____	_____
_____	_____
_____	_____
_____	_____
_____	_____
_____	_____
_____	_____

TEST YOUR KNOWLEDGE

Section A

Divide and define the following terms.

1. Keratoplasty _repair of the cornea_
2. Cerebral meningitis _inflamation of the cerebral meninges_
3. Neurasthenia _weak nerves_
4. Encephaloma _tumor in the brain_
5. Retinopathy _disease of the retina_
6. Schizophrenia _condition of splitting of the mind_
7. Myelogram _record of muscle_
8. Psychology _study of the mind_
9. Myringoscope _instrument used to examine the eardrum_
10. Periophthalmic _pertaining to around the eye_
11. Neurosis _condition of (often abnormal) nerves_
12. Intraventricular _pertaining to within the ventricle_
13. Cerebrospinal _____
14. Anencephalic _pertaining to without a brain_
15. Conjunctivitis _inflammation of the conjunctiva_

Section B

Construct terms for the following definitions.

1. Infection of the meninges _mening itis_
2. Pertaining to the pons and the cerebellum _____
3. Pain in the ear _____
4. Herniation of the meninges _meningocele_
5. Deficiency of tears _lacro penic_
6. Pertaining to the medulla _____
7. Destruction of nerves _neurolysis_
8. Disease of the spinal cord _pathy_
9. Specialist in the study of nerves _ologist_
10. Incision into the eardrum _tomy_

72

Section C

Complete the following definitions.

1. Pont/o/medull/ary   pertaining to the _____ and _MARROW_
2. Peri/ocul/ar   around the _EYE_
3. Par/ot/id gland   gland alongside the _____
4. Tympan/o/sclerosis   hardening of the _EARdrum_
5. Psych/o/somat/ic   pertaining to _mind & body_ and body
6. Lacrim/ase   enzyme in the _tEArs_
7. Ot/o/logist   specialist in the _study of EArs_
8. Poli/o/myel/itis   inflammation of the gray (matter) of the _SpinAl cord_
9. Neur/o/rrhaphy   suturing of a _nErvE_
10. Ophthalm/o/my/itis   inflammation of the muscles of the _EyE_

Section D

Complete the following terms.

1. _____lAcrimo_ cystitis   inflammation of the tear sac
2. _____rEtino_scopy   examination of the retina
3. _____ graphy   recording of the ventricles
4. _____ cranial   pertaining to external ear and skull
5. _____ pyorrhea   flow of pus from the ear
6. Micr_____y   abnormally small brain
7. _____ al fluid   pertaining to cerebrum and spinal cord
8. _____ malacia   softening of the meninges
9. _____ therapy   treatment of nerve (disorders)
10. _____ atrophia   atrophy of a nerve

Answers to Lesson 10—page 220

On the following pages are:

1. Unlabeled diagrams of the brain, ear, and eye. On each label line, write in the name of the part.

2. A diagram of the spinal nerves and some of their branches. Practice using your terminology by seeing how many of these names you can analyze.

Write each term or combining form on the appropriate label line.
Cerebello- (use twice)   Myelo- (use twice)
Cerebro- (use twice)   Oculo-
Hypo-   Olfactory
Longitudinal   Optic
Mamm-   Ponto- (use twice)
Medullo- (use twice)   Ventriculo-
Mes-

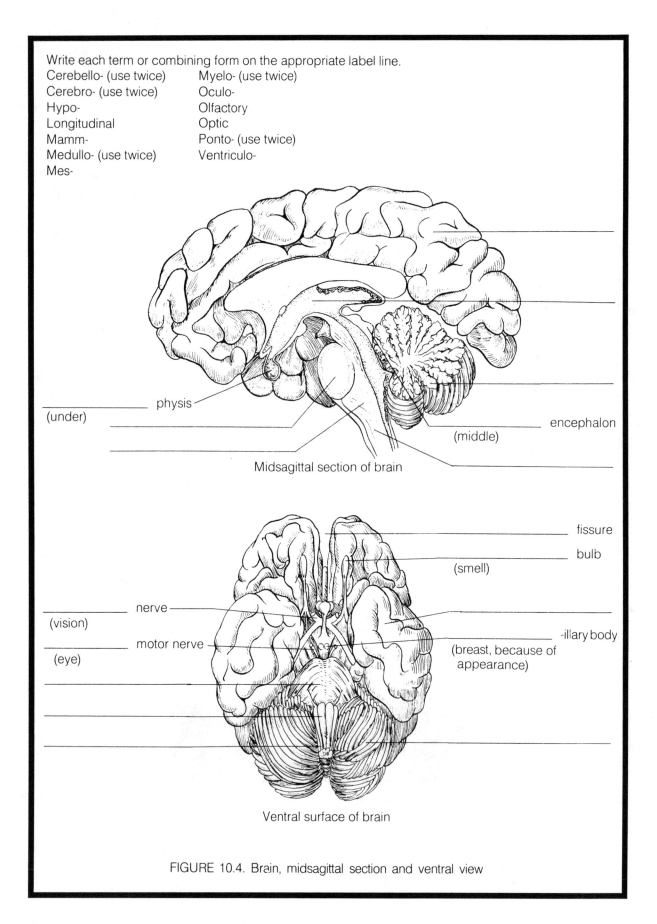

_____ physis

(under)

_____ encephalon

(middle)

Midsagittal section of brain

_____ fissure

_____ bulb

(smell)

nerve _____

(vision)

motor nerve _____

(eye)

-illary body

(breast, because of appearance)

Ventral surface of brain

FIGURE 10.4. Brain, midsagittal section and ventral view

Write each term or combining form on the appropriate label line.
Acoustic (use twice)
Auditory (use twice)
Auriculo-
Cochleo-
External
Ossicles
Tympano-, myringo-

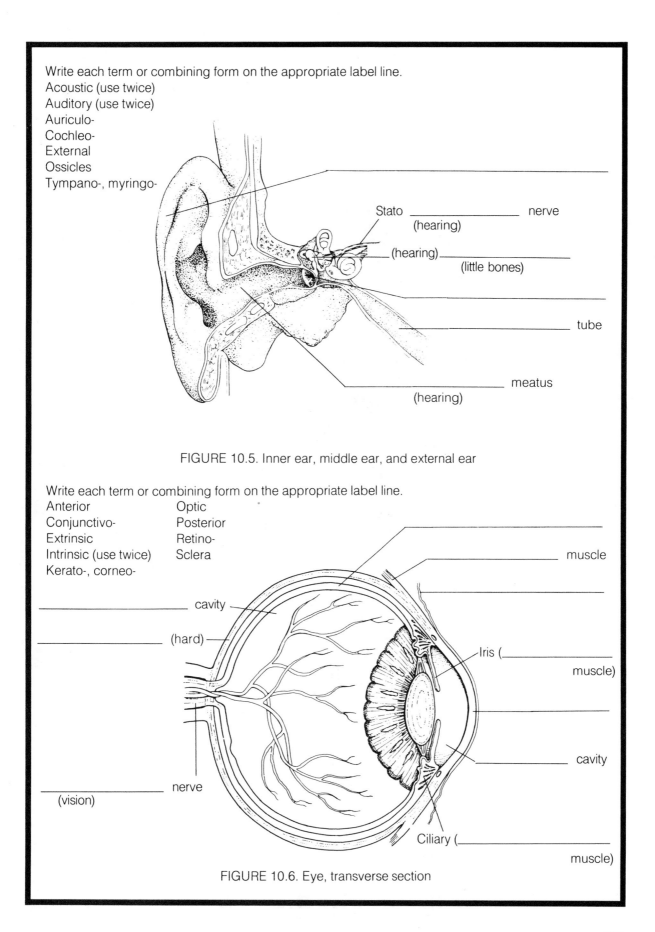

Stato _____ nerve
(hearing)

_____ (hearing) _____
(little bones)

_____ tube

_____ meatus
(hearing)

FIGURE 10.5. Inner ear, middle ear, and external ear

Write each term or combining form on the appropriate label line.
Anterior   Optic
Conjunctivo-   Posterior
Extrinsic   Retino-
Intrinsic (use twice) Sclera
Kerato-, corneo-

_____ muscle

_____ cavity

_____ (hard)

Iris (_____ muscle)

_____ cavity

_____ nerve
(vision)

Ciliary (_____ muscle)

FIGURE 10.6. Eye, transverse section

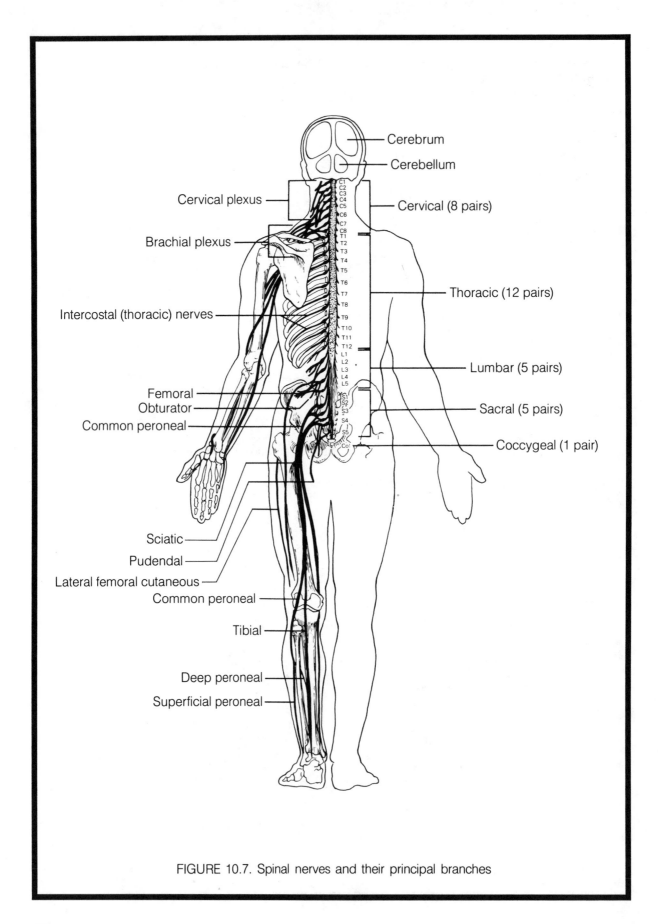

Cerebrum

Cerebellum

Cervical plexus

Cervical (8 pairs)

Brachial plexus

Thoracic (12 pairs)

Intercostal (thoracic) nerves

Lumbar (5 pairs)

Femoral

Obturator

Sacral (5 pairs)

Common peroneal

Coccygeal (1 pair)

Sciatic

Pudendal

Lateral femoral cutaneous

Common peroneal

Tibial

Deep peroneal

Superficial peroneal

FIGURE 10.7. Spinal nerves and their principal branches

76

Variations on the Theme 1
Diminutives, Spelling, Nouns and Adjectives

Unfortunately, not all terms are built from obvious parts. This lesson and Lesson 13 present some of the items you must watch for in your word study.

1. Diminutives (from Latin, meaning to make small)
   If a suffix contains the letter l, the diminutive form is indicated and the modifier *small* or *little* is used in the translation.
   For example:

   corpus = body   corpuscle = little body

   ped = foot   peduncle = little foot

   What is the meaning of each of the following?

   arteriole _little artery_____

   venule _little vein_____

   bronchiole _little bronchi_____

2. Spelling
   The importance of correct spelling cannot be overemphasized. Be aware of spelling as you learn words, and drill yourself if necessary. Following are some aspects of spelling that may help you.

   a. Sometimes when elements are combined into words the spelling must be changed to avoid awkwardness. For example:

      In uremia, -em- is all that is left of hemo- (meaning blood).

      Symphysis is from syn (meaning with) and physis (meaning grow).

      Collateral is from con (meaning together) and lateral (meaning side).

   In the latter two, the n is softened to blend with the following word root.

   b. When a prefix ending in o or a is combined with a word root beginning with the same vowel, the spelling is handled in various ways. For example:

      In micr/ophthalmia and hyp/onychium the o is dropped from the prefix and only the o of the word root is used.

      In retro-ocular and intra-abdominal the problem is solved with a hyphen.

      In microorganism both o's are used, but they are pronounced separately.

   c. Some terms appear to be difficult to divide because there are two possibilities for the prefix. For example:

      In analgesia and anaerobic, an- is the prefix, not ana-.

      In diagnosis, dia- is the prefix (-gnosis meaning knowledge), but in diarthric, di- (meaning two) is the prefix.

   Also note that occasionally a prefix is used between two word roots, as in my/a/sthenia (without muscle strength).

d. In some cases an error in only one letter creates an entirely different word or word element. For example:

ileum/ilium

ante-/anti-

hemi-/hemo-

e. Another common error that causes confusion is to insert or leave out one letter when analyzing or constructing a word. For example:

cyto-/cysto-

pyo-/pyro-

To avoid errors like those noted in **d** and **e**, study the list of frequently confused word elements given with Review Test 2.

3. One word root with two meanings

A problem arises when the same English word root has two different meanings. For example:

The word roots metr- and my- are each derived from two different Greek words.

metr- = uterus, as in endometrium

metr- = measure, as in metric

my- = muscle, as in myocardium

my- = shut, as in myopia

The word root myel- means either bone marrow or spinal cord. (Here it is easy to see the reason for the two meanings. The spinal cord is soft tissue within the vertebral column, so the similarity to the soft tissue inside a single bone is apparent).

In all such cases the solution is to try all possibilities until the meaning seems correct in the context in which the word is used.

4. Nouns and adjectives (noun, from Latin, meaning to name; adjective, from Latin, meaning to add to)

In some cases a noun may be converted to an adjective by adding a suffix meaning *pertaining to*. The reverse process would, of course, convert an adjective to a noun. For example:

Noun	Adjective
stethoscope	stethoscopic
hemophilia	hemophiliac
cerebrum	cerebral

In other cases, a -tic suffix accomplishes the conversion to an adjective. For example:

Noun	Adjective
necrosis	necrotic
pepsia	peptic
anorexia	anorectic

Watch for other techniques used for these conversions. If you are unfamiliar with the examples used, look up the word elements in the glossary-index.

Note: Although you should be on the lookout for the factors of construction mentioned in this lesson, do not be overly concerned about them now. As you use terminology in future courses and in your profession you will become familiar with the variations and eventually use and recognize them easily.

TEST YOUR KNOWLEDGE

1. What letter in a suffix indicates the diminutive? ___L___

2. How do you decide the proper way to divide a term into its elements when there is more than one possibility?

   _____

3. If a word root in a term has two meanings, how do you decide which one is correct? _____

   _____

4. What book do you use if you are puzzled about divisions or definitions? _____

5. Change the following nouns to adjectives and give the meaning of both forms.

Noun	Meaning	Adjective	Pertaining to
a. Neurosis	Abnormal nerve condition	neurotic	nerves
b. Schizophrenia	condition of split mind	schizophrenic	split mind
c. Microscope	instrument to examine sm. things	microscopic	examination of sm things
d. Arthritis	inflammation of joints	arthritic	inflammed joints
e. Meter	instrument to measure	metric	measure
f. Hyperplasia	more than normal formation ~~tocc~~	hyperplastic	
g. Syndactyly (digits) (with together)	with digits together	syndactylic	
h. Carcinogen	cancer producing	carcinogenic	
i. Osteolysis	decomposition of bone	osteolytic	
j. Cranium	head skull	cranial	

6. Change the following adjectives to nouns and give the meaning of both forms.

Adjective	Pertaining to	Noun	Meaning
a. Antiseptic	against infections		
b. Pubic	pubis	pubus	
c. Genetic	~~place of origin~~ formation		
d. Auricular	ear		
e. Analgesic	sensation of pain		
f. Medullary	marrow		
g. Dyspeptic	(painful) bad digestion		
h. Biological	study of life	biology	
i. Spastic	spasm		
j. Narcotic	numbness		

Answers to Lesson 11—page 221

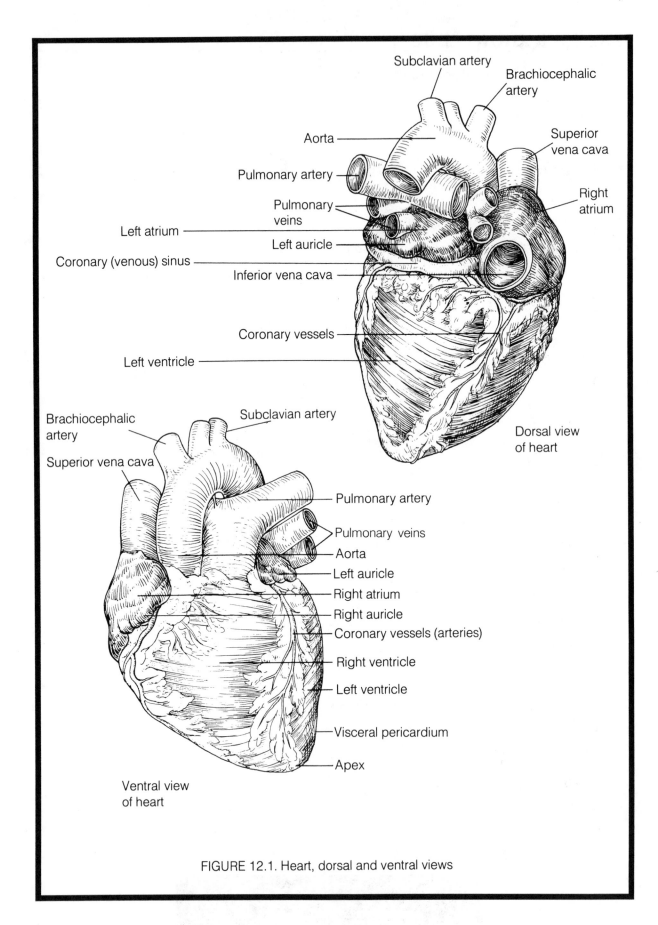

Subclavian artery

Brachiocephalic artery

Aorta

Pulmonary artery

Superior vena cava

Pulmonary veins

Right atrium

Left atrium

Left auricle

Coronary (venous) sinus

Inferior vena cava

Coronary vessels

Left ventricle

Dorsal view of heart

Brachiocephalic artery

Subclavian artery

Superior vena cava

Pulmonary artery

Pulmonary veins

Aorta

Left auricle

Right atrium

Right auricle

Coronary vessels (arteries)

Right ventricle

Left ventricle

Visceral pericardium

Apex

Ventral view of heart

FIGURE 12.1. Heart, dorsal and ventral views

Circulatory System

Circulatory: from Latin, meaning forming a circle

A transportation system is vital to all body cells, since they require nutrients and produce waste and are located at some distance from the organs that handle these functions. The circulatory system is responsible for transporting these substances, as well as enzymes and hormones. Blood travels in a closed circuit consisting of the *heart, arteries, capillaries, and veins.* Each complete trip around the body includes passage through the lungs for gas exchange.

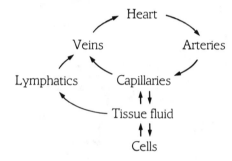

The capillary walls are extremely thin, permitting fluid to pass in and out of the blood as substances are exchanged with the cells. The heart is the muscular pump that maintains the flow of blood. The arteries and veins complete the circuit. A network of *lymphatic vessels* returns to the blood a portion of the tissue fluid that has supplied the cells. On its way to the veins, this *lymph* is filtered through one or more lymph nodes for the removal of bacteria and other potentially harmful particles.

The human heart has four chambers, with the right and left sides separated to prevent the mixing of high oxygen and low oxygen blood. This separation maintains high enough levels of oxygen in the blood to permit the rate of heat production by cells that is necessary to keep body temperature constant. The upper chambers, called *atria,* receive blood from the veins and pass it on to the *ventricles,* which pump it into the arteries. A *valve* at the exit of each chamber prevents the backflow of blood.

Blood is composed of a liquid *plasma* and several types of cells known as *erythrocytes* (red blood cells, which carry oxygen), *leukocytes* (white blood cells, which fight infection), and *thrombocytes* (platelets, which play a role in clotting). If blood is allowed to clot and the clot is then removed, the remaining fluid is *serum.* Serum is a useful substance because it contains the protein antibodies that confer immunity on a specific basis. The *thymus* gland and lymph nodes are concerned with the production of these antibodies. The *spleen* stores blood and performs other blood-related functions.

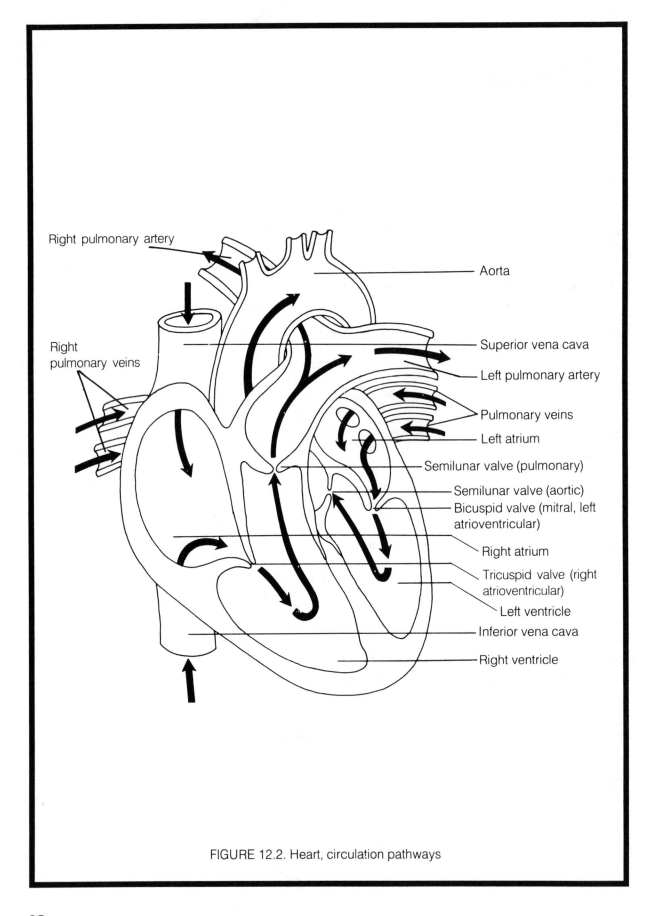

Right pulmonary artery

Right pulmonary veins

Aorta

Superior vena cava

Left pulmonary artery

Pulmonary veins

Left atrium

Semilunar valve (pulmonary)

Semilunar valve (aortic)

Bicuspid valve (mitral, left atrioventricular)

Right atrium

Tricuspid valve (right atrioventricular)

Left ventricle

Inferior vena cava

Right ventricle

FIGURE 12.2. Heart, circulation pathways

		Aids to Learning	
Combining Form	**Anatomical Use**	**Illustrative Words**	**Literal Meaning**
cardio- (KAR-dē-ō)	heart	electrocardiogram	
atrio- (Ā-trē-ō)	atrium	atrioventricular	corridor
ventriculo- (ven-TRIK-ū-lō)	ventricle		little belly
auriculo- (aw-RIK-ū-lō)	auricular appendage of atrial wall		little ear
corono- (KAW-rō-nō)	arteries of heart	coronary, coronation	crown
mitro- (MĪ-trō)	mitral valve		bishop's hat
angio-, vaso- (AN-jē-ō) (VAS-ō)	vessel	angiogram, vascular	
arterio- (ar-TĒ-rē-ō)	artery	arteriosclerosis	
sphygmo-, sphyx- (SFIG-mō) (sfiks)	pulse	asphyxiate, sphygmometer	
phlebo-, veno- (FLEB-ō) (VĒ-nō)	vein	phlebitis, venous	
capillaro- (KAP-i-lār-ō)	capillary		little hair
spleno- (SPLĒ-nō)	spleen		
thymo- (THĪ-mō)	thymus gland		
hemo-, hema-, (HĒ-mō) (HĒM-a) **hemato-** (HĒM-a-tō)	blood	hemorrhoid, hematoma	
lympho- (LIM-fō)	lymph		water

		Aids to Learning	
Combining Form	Anatomical Use	Illustrative Words	Literal Meaning
plasmo- (PLAZ-mō)	plasma	plasmotherapy	something formed
sero- (SĒ-rō)	serum	serological	whey

WORDS USING THESE ELEMENTS

Record words given in class or encountered in your reading.

Word	Meaning

ic, ac, ascary, ory, a|ea|, ous

TEST YOUR KNOWLEDGE

Section A

Divide and define the following terms.

1. Hemorrhage _Extreme Flow of ~~rupture~~ blood (vessel)_
2. Splenomegaly _enlargement of the spleen_
3. Cardiovascular _pertaining to ~~vessels of the~~ heart & VESSELS_
4. Angiogram _recording of vessels_

5. Coronary _pertaining to arteries of the heart_

6. Phlebitis _inflammation of vein_

7. Atrioventricular _pertaining to atrium & ventricle_

8. Arteriole _small artery_

9. Vasodilatation _dilation of the vessel_

10. Hematuria _condition of urine in the blood_   _blood in the urine_

11. Endocarditis _inflammation inside the heart_

12. Lymphangitis _inflammation of lymph vessel_

13. Serology _study of serum_

14. Thymolytic _pertaining to destruction of the thymus gland_

15. Hematopoiesis _formation of blood_

16. Splenorrhagia _~~rupture~~ of spleen_ EXTREME flow

17. Hemangioma _tumor in the blood vessel_

18. Myocardial _pertaining to heart muscle_

19. Serous _full of serum_   _pertaining to serum_

20. Phlebectasia _dilitation of the vein_

Section B

Construct terms for the following definitions.

1. Dilatation of the heart _cardioectasis_   _CARDIOECTASIA_

2. Between the atria _interatrial_

3. Tumor in a vessel _angioma_

4. Hardening of the arteries _arteriosclerosis_

5. Instrument to measure the pulse _sphyxometer_   _sphygmometer_

6. Removal of the spleen _splenectomy_

7. Disease of the heart _cardiopathy_

8. Destruction of blood _hematolysis_   _hemolysis_

9. Swelling related to lymph _lymphedema_

10. Stricture of the mitral valve _mitrostenosis_

Section C

Complete the following definitions.

1. A/sphyxia   without a _pulse_

2. Lymph/aden/oma   tumor of a _lymph_ gland

3. Ser/o/therapy   treatment with _serum_

4. Vas/o/pressin   hormone that increases pressure in _vessels_

5. Thymo/tox/ic   poisonous to the _thymus gland_

6. Angi/o/tripsy   crushing of a _vessel_

7. Splen/odynia   pain in the _spleen_

8. Peri/card/ium   (membrane) around the _heart_

9. Hemat/oma   _____ _blood_ _____ tumor

10. Capillar/o/pathy   disease of _capillaries_

Section D

Complete the following terms.

1. _____ _cardio_ rrhexis   rupture of the heart

2. _____ _plasma_ apheresis   removal of plasma

3. _____ _Angio_ / _vaso_ spasm   spasm of a vessel

4. _coronary_ _corono-_ occlusion   blockage of heart arteries

5. Thrombo_____ _ven_ _phleb_ itis   inflammation of veins with clotting

6. _____ _hemato_ coelia   blood in the body cavity

7. _____ _thymo_ sin   hormone made in thymus

8. _____ _arterio_ sclerosis   hardening of arteries

9. _____ _cardio_ megaly   enlargement of heart

10. _____ _hemato_ emesis   vomiting of blood

Answers to Lesson 12—page 222

On the following pages are:

1. Diagrams of the heart. On each label line. write in the name of the part.

2. Diagrams of the principal arteries and veins of the body. Practice using your terminology by seeing how many of the names you can analyze.

Write each term or combining form on the appropriate label line.

Atrio- (use three times)   Left (use twice)   Superior (use twice)
Auriculo- (use three times)   Right (use twice)   Ventriculo- (use four times)
Brachiocephalic (use twice)   Subclavian (use twice)   Visceral pericardium
Corono- (use twice)
Inferior

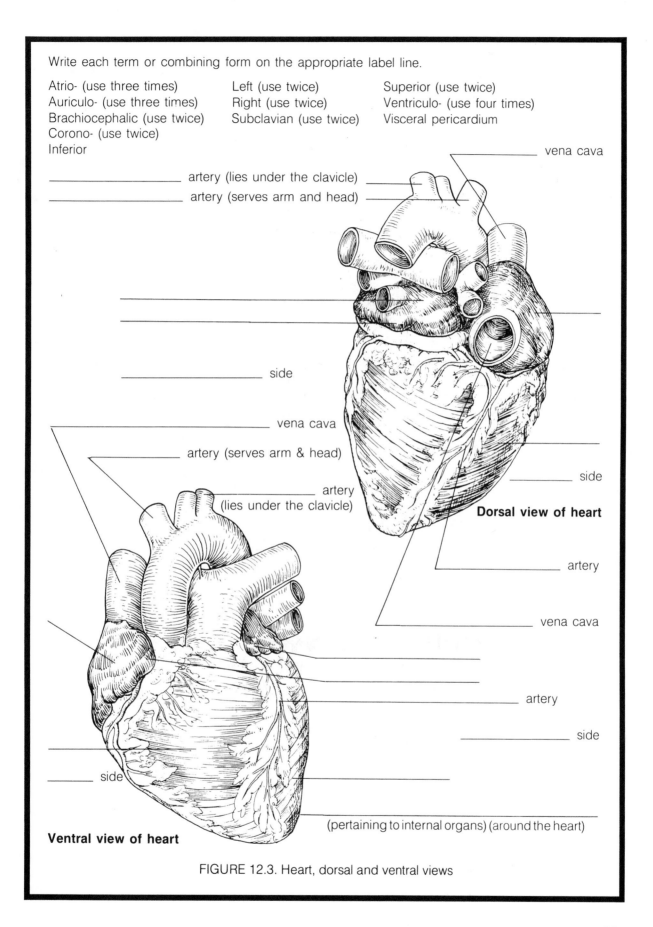

_____ vena cava

_____ artery (lies under the clavicle)
_____ artery (serves arm and head)

_____ side

_____ vena cava

_____ artery (serves arm & head)

_____ artery
(lies under the clavicle)

_____ side

Dorsal view of heart

_____ artery

_____ vena cava

_____ artery

_____ side

_____ side

Ventral view of heart

(pertaining to internal organs) (around the heart)

FIGURE 12.3. Heart, dorsal and ventral views

87

Write each term or combining form on the appropriate label line.

Atrio- (use twice)
Atrioventricular (use twice)
Inferior
Left
Mitro-
Right
Superior
Ventriculo- (use twice)

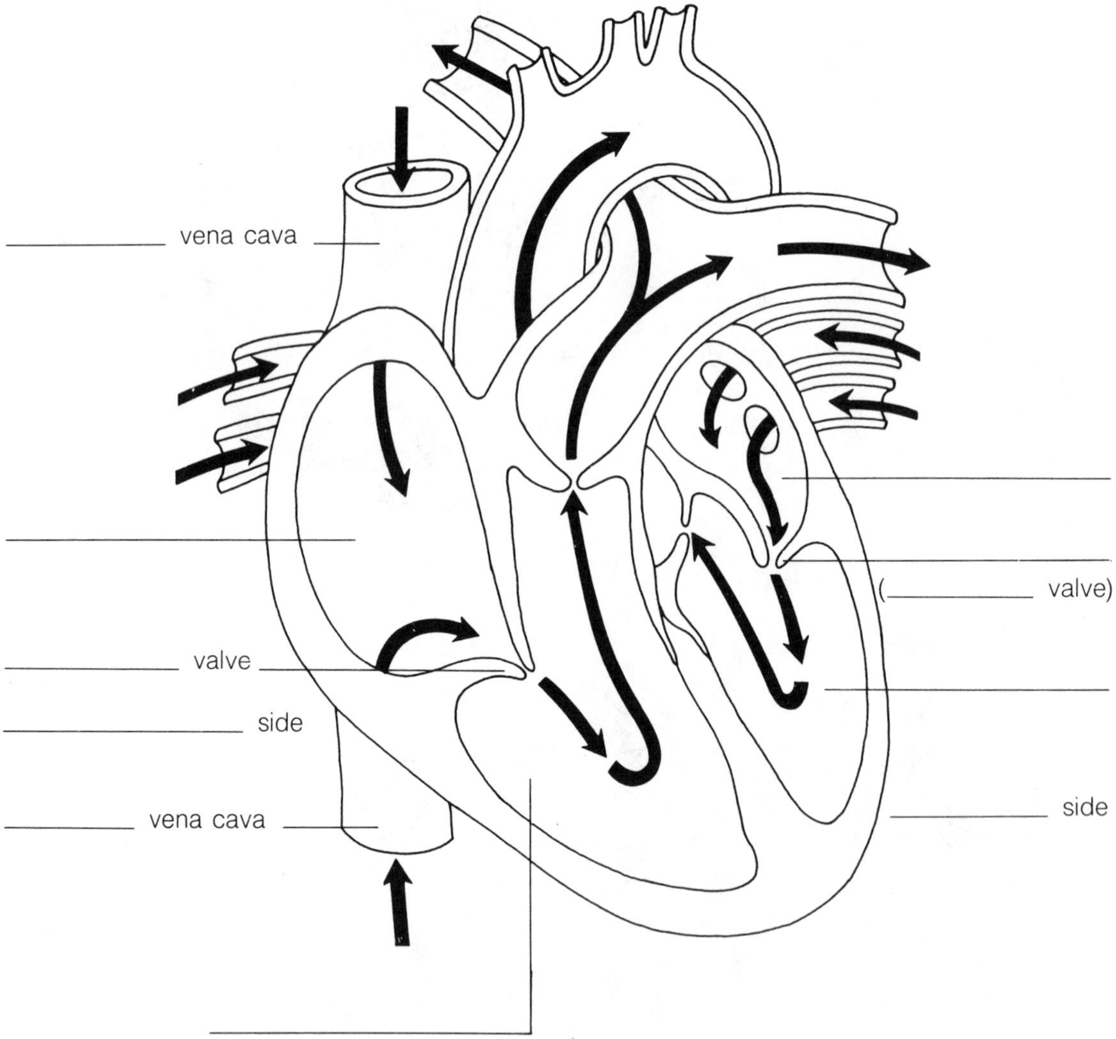

_____ vena cava

_____

valve _____

_____ side

_____ vena cava

(_____ valve)

_____ side

FIGURE 12.4. Heart, circulation pathways

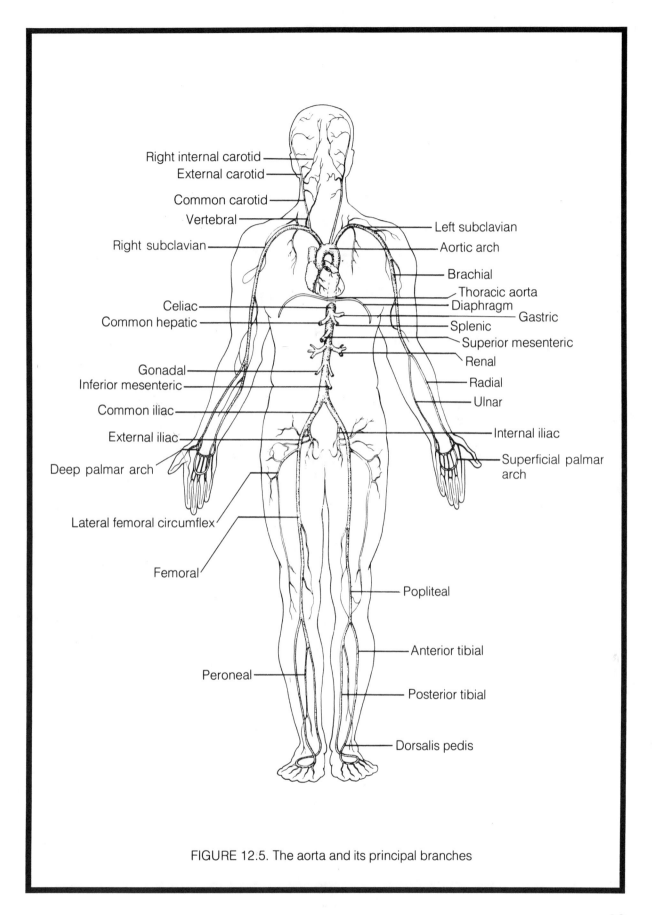

FIGURE 12.5. The aorta and its principal branches

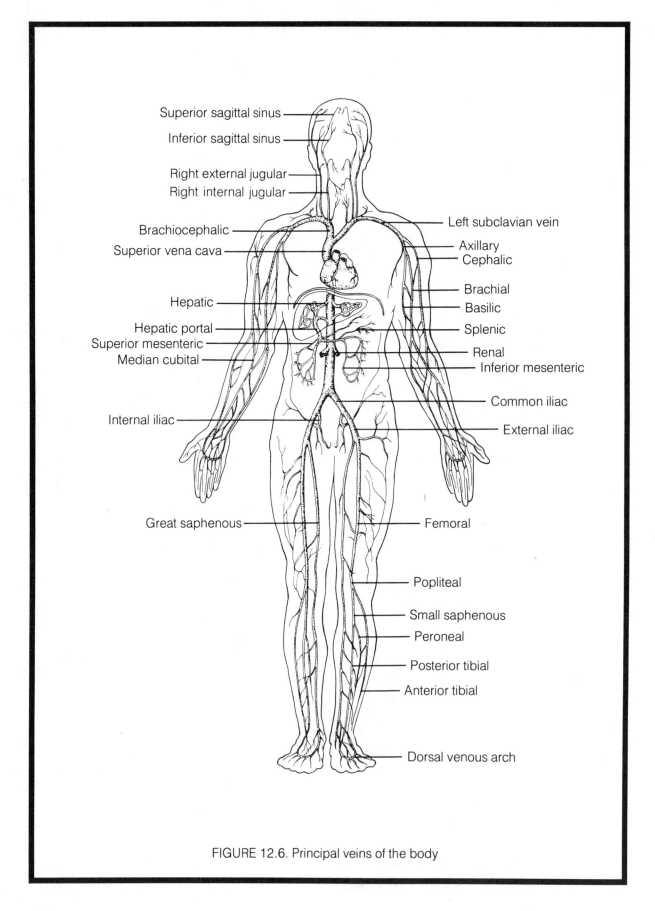

Superior sagittal sinus

Inferior sagittal sinus

Right external jugular
Right internal jugular

Left subclavian vein

Brachiocephalic
Superior vena cava

Axillary
Cephalic

Brachial

Hepatic

Basilic

Hepatic portal
Superior mesenteric
Median cubital

Splenic

Renal
Inferior mesenteric

Common iliac

Internal iliac

External iliac

Great saphenous

Femoral

Popliteal

Small saphenous

Peroneal

Posterior tibial

Anterior tibial

Dorsal venous arch

FIGURE 12.6. Principal veins of the body

TERMINOLOGY SEARCH 2: A DRUG FLYER

For each drug it produces, a pharmaceutical company prepares a detailed information sheet that is packaged with the drug. Here is an example.

CAUTION: Federal law prohibits dispensing without prescription.

BEFORE USING INDERAL (PROPRANOLOL HYDROCHLORIDE), THE PHYSICIAN SHOULD BE THOROUGHLY FAMILIAR WITH THE BASIC CONCEPT OF ADRENERGIC RECEPTORS (ALPHA AND BETA), AND THE PHARMACOLOGY OF THIS DRUG.

DESCRIPTION

Chemical name: 1-(Isopropylamino)-3-(1-naphthyloxy)-2-propanol hydrochloride

Structural formula:

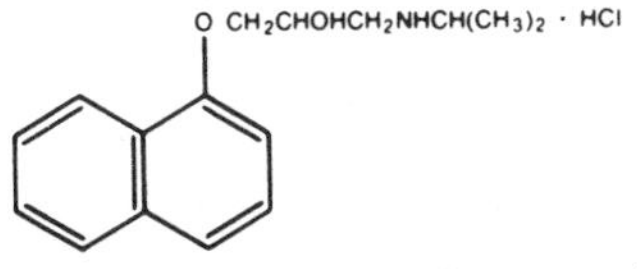
O CH₂CHOHCH₂NHCH(CH₃)₂ · HCl

INDERAL (propranolol hydrochloride) is a stable, colorless, crystalline solid with a melting point of about 164° C. It is readily soluble in water and ethanol and insoluble in non-polar solvents.

ACTIONS

INDERAL is a beta-adrenergic receptor blocking drug, possessing no other autonomic nervous system activity. It specifically competes with beta-adrenergic receptor stimulating agents for available beta receptor sites. When access to beta receptor sites is blocked by INDERAL, the chronotropic, inotropic, and vasodilator responses to beta-adrenergic stimulation are decreased proportionately.

Propranolol is almost completely absorbed from the gastrointestinal tract, but a portion is immediately bound by the liver. Peak effect occurs in one to one and one-half hours. The biologic half-life is approximately two to three hours. Propranolol is not significantly dialyzable. There is no simple correlation between dose or plasma level and therapeutic effect, and the dose-sensitivity range as observed in clinical practice is wide. The principal reason for this is that sympathetic tone varies widely between individuals. Since there is no reliable test to estimate sympathetic tone or to determine whether total beta blockade has been achieved, proper dosage requires titration.

The mechanism of the antihypertensive and antimigraine effects of INDERAL have not been established. Among the factors that may be involved in the antihypertensive action are (1) decreased cardiac output, (2) inhibition of renin release by the kidneys, and (3) diminution of tonic sympathetic nerve outflow from vasomotor centers in the brain. The antimigraine effect may be due to inhibition of vasodilation or to the fact that beta-adrenergic receptors have been demonstrated in the pial vessels of the brain and that arteriolar spasms over the cortex can be inhibited with INDERAL.

Propranolol hydrochloride decreases heart rate, cardiac output, and blood pressure. Although total peripheral vascular resistance may increase initially, it readjusts to the pretreatment level, or lower, with chronic usage. Earlier studies indicate that plasma volume remains unchanged or may decrease. However, there are certain more recent studies suggesting that in the absence of sodium restriction, plasma volume may increase.

Beta receptor blockade is useful in conditions in which, because of pathologic or functional changes, sympathetic activity is excessive or inappropriate and detrimental to the patient. But there are also situations in which sympathetic stimulation is vital. For example, in patients with severely damaged hearts, adequate ventricular function is maintained by virtue of sympathetic drive which should be preserved. In the presence of AV block, beta blockade may prevent the necessary facilitating effect of sympathetic activity on conduction. Beta blockade results in bronchial constriction by interfering with adrenergic bronchodilator activity which should be preserved in patients subject to bronchospasm.

The proper objective of beta blockade therapy is to decrease adverse sympathetic stimulation but not to the degree that may impair necessary sympathetic support.

Propranolol exerts its antiarrhythmic effects in concentrations associated with beta-adrenergic blockade and this appears to be its principal antiarrhythmic mechanism of action. The membrane effect also plays a role, particularly, some authorities believe, in digitalis-induced arrhythmias. Beta-adrenergic blockade is of unique importance in the management of arrhythmias due to increased levels of circulating catecholamines or enhanced sensitivity of the heart to catecholamines (arrhythmias associated with pheochromocytoma, thyrotoxicosis, exercise).

In dosages greater than required for beta blockade, INDERAL also exerts a quinidine-like or anesthetic-like membrane action which affects the cardiac action potential and depresses cardiac function.

Propranolol may reduce the oxygen requirement of the heart at any given level of effort by blocking catecholamine-induced increases in heart rate, systolic blood pressure, and the velocity and extent of myocardial contraction. On the other hand, propranolol may increase oxygen requirements by increasing left ventricular fiber length, end diastolic pressure, and systolic ejection period.

If the net physiologic effect of beta-adrenergic blockade in angina is advantageous, it would be expected to manifest itself during exercise by delayed onset of pain due to decreased oxygen requirement.

INDICATIONS

Hypertension

INDERAL is indicated in the management of hypertension. It is usually used in combination with other drugs, particularly a thiazide diuretic. INDERAL is not indicated for treatment of hypertensive emergencies.

Angina Pectoris Due to Coronary Atherosclerosis

The initial treatment of angina pectoris involves weight control, rest, cessation of smoking, use of sublingual nitroglycerin, and avoidance of precipitating circumstances. INDERAL is indicated in selected patients with moderate to severe angina pectoris who have not responded to these conventional measures. Propranolol should not be used in patients with angina which occurs only with considerable effort or with infrequent precipitating factors.

INDERAL exerts both favorable and unfavorable effects, the preponderance of which may be beneficial. (See ACTIONS Section.) INDERAL should not be continued unless there is reduced pain or increased work capacity.

Because of the potential for adverse results, treatment should be carefully monitored. The patient should also be reevaluated periodically since the dosage requirement and the need to continue INDERAL may be altered by clinical exacerbations or remissions. (See DOSAGE AND ADMINISTRATION.)

Additional studies of the effects of INDERAL in angina pectoris patients are in progress to better evaluate and define the proper role of INDERAL in this condition.

Cardiac Arrhythmias

1.) Supraventricular arrhythmias
   a) Paroxysmal atrial tachycardias, particularly those arrhythmias induced by catecholamines or digitalis or associated with the Wolff-Parkinson-White syndrome. (See W-P-W under WARNINGS.)
   b) Persistent sinus tachycardia which is noncompensatory and impairs the well-being of the patient.
   c) Tachycardias and arrhythmias due to thyrotoxicosis when causing distress or increased hazard and when immediate effect is necessary as adjunctive, short term (2-4 weeks) therapy. May be used with, but not in place of, specific therapy. (See Thyrotoxicosis under WARNINGS.)
   d) Persistent atrial extrasystoles which impair the well-being of the patient and do not respond to conventional measures.
   e) Atrial flutter and fibrillation when ventricular rate cannot be controlled by digitalis alone, or when digitalis is contraindicated.

2.) Ventricular tachycardias

   Ventricular arrhythmias do not respond to propranolol as predictably as do the supraventricular arrhythmias.
   a) Ventricular tachycardias

      With the exception of those induced by catecholamines or digitalis, INDERAL is not the drug of first choice. In critical situations when cardioversion technics or other drugs are not indicated or are not effective, INDERAL may be considered. If, after consideration of the risks involved, INDERAL is used, it should be given intravenously in low dosage and very slowly. (See DOSAGE AND ADMINISTRATION.) *Care in the administration of* INDERAL *with constant electrocardiographic monitoring is essential as the failing heart requires some sympathetic drive for maintenance of myocardial tone.*
   b) Persistent premature ventricular extrasystoles which do not respond to conventional measures and impair the well-being of the patient.

3.) Tachyarrhythmias of digitalis intoxication

   If digitalis-induced tachyarrhythmias persist following discontinuance of digitalis and correction of electrolyte abnormalities, they are usually reversible with *oral* INDERAL. Severe bradycardia may occur. (See OVERDOSAGE OR EXAGGERATED RESPONSE.)

   Intravenous propranolol hydrochloride is reserved for life-threatening arrhythmias. Temporary maintenance with oral therapy may be indicated. (See DOSAGE AND ADMINISTRATION.)

4.) Resistant tachyarrhythmias due to excessive catecholamine action during anesthesia

   Tachyarrhythmias due to excessive catecholamine action during anesthesia may sometimes arise because of release of endogenous catecholamines or administration of catecholamines. When usual measures fail in such arrhythmias, INDERAL may be given intravenously to abolish them. All general inhalation anesthetics produce some degree of myocardial depression. Therefore, when INDERAL is used to treat arrhythmias during anesthesia, it should be used with extreme caution and constant ECG and central venous pressure monitoring. (See WARNINGS.)

Migraine

INDERAL is indicated for the prophylaxis of common migraine headache. The efficacy of INDERAL in the treatment of a migraine attack that has already started has not been established and INDERAL is not indicated for such use.

Vascular headaches of the migraine type are often familial, are recurrent, and vary widely in frequency, duration, and intensity. The attacks are commonly unilateral in onset, and are usually associated with anorexia, and sometimes nausea and vomiting. In females, these headaches often occur premenstrually or early during the menses. Migraine attacks are sometimes preceded by, or associated with, conspicuous sensory, motor, and mood disturbances, but common migraine usually occurs without striking prodromes, and is less often unilateral.

Hypertrophic Subaortic Stenosis

INDERAL is useful in the management of hypertrophic subaortic stenosis, especially for treatment of exertional or other stress-induced angina, palpitations, and syncope. INDERAL also improves exercise performance. The effectiveness of INDERAL in this disease appears to be due to a reduction of the elevated outflow pressure gradient which is exacerbated by beta receptor stimulation. Clinical improvement may be temporary.

Pheochromocytoma

After primary treatment with an alpha-adrenergic blocking agent has been instituted, INDERAL may be useful as *adjunctive* therapy if the control of tachycardia becomes necessary before or during surgery.

It is hazardous to use INDERAL unless alpha-adrenergic blocking drugs are already in use, since this would predispose to serious blood pressure elevation. Blocking only the peripheral dilator (beta) action of epinephrine leaves its constrictor (alpha) action unopposed.

In the event of hemorrhage or shock, there is a disadvantage in having both beta and alpha blockade since the combination prevents the increase in heart rate and peripheral vasoconstriction needed to maintain blood pressure.

With inoperable or metastatic pheochromocytoma, INDERAL may be useful as an adjunct to the management of symptoms due to excessive beta receptor stimulation.

CONTRAINDICATIONS

INDERAL is contraindicated in: 1) bronchial asthma; 2) allergic rhinitis during the pollen season; 3) sinus bradycardia and greater than first degree block; 4) cardiogenic shock; 5) right ventricular failure secondary to pulmonary hypertension; 6) congestive heart failure (see WARNINGS) unless the failure is secondary to a tachyarrhythmia treatable with INDERAL; 7) in patients on adrenergic-augmenting psychotropic drugs (including MAO inhibitors), and during the two week withdrawal period from such drugs.

WARNINGS

CARDIAC FAILURE: Sympathetic stimulation is a vital component supporting circulatory function in congestive heart failure, and inhibition with beta-blockade always carries the potential hazard of further depressing myocardial contractility and precipitating cardiac failure. INDERAL acts selectively without abolishing the inotropic action of digitalis on the heart muscle (*i.e.*, that of supporting the strength of myocardial contractions). In patients already receiving digitalis, the positive inotropic action of digitalis may be reduced by INDERAL's negative inotropic effect. The effects of INDERAL and digitalis are additive in depressing AV conduction.

IN PATIENTS WITHOUT A HISTORY OF CARDIAC FAILURE, continued depression of the myocardium over a period of time can, in some cases, lead to cardiac failure. In rare instances, this has been observed during INDERAL therapy. Therefore, at the first sign or symptom of impending cardiac failure, patients should be fully digitalized and/or given a diuretic, and the response observed closely: a) if cardiac failure continues, despite adequate digitalization and diuretic therapy, INDERAL therapy should be immediately withdrawn; b) if tachyarrhythmia is being controlled, patients should be maintained on combined therapy and the patient closely followed until threat of cardiac failure is over.

IN PATIENTS WITH ANGINA PECTORIS, there have been reports of exacerbation of angina and, in some cases, myocardial infarction, following abrupt discontinuation of INDERAL therapy. Therefore, when discontinuance of INDERAL is planned the dosage should be gradually reduced and the patient carefully monitored. In addition, when INDERAL is prescribed for angina pectoris, the patient should be cautioned against interruption or cessation of therapy without the physician's advice. If INDERAL therapy is interrupted and exacerbation of angina occurs, it usually is advisable to reinstitute INDERAL therapy and take other measures appropriate for the management of unstable angina pectoris. Since coronary artery disease may be unrecognized, it may be prudent to follow the above advice in patients considered at risk of having occult atherosclerotic heart disease, who are given propranolol for other indications.

IN PATIENTS WITH THYROTOXICOSIS, possible deleterious effects from long term use have not been adequately appraised. Special consideration should be given to propranolol's potential for aggravating congestive heart failure. Propranolol may mask the clinical signs of developing or continuing hyperthyroidism or complications and give a false impression of improvement. Therefore, abrupt withdrawal of propranolol may be followed by an exacerbation of symptoms of hyperthyroidism, including thyroid storm. This is another reason for withdrawing propranolol slowly. Propranolol does not distort thyroid function tests.

IN PATIENTS WITH WOLFF-PARKINSON-WHITE SYNDROME, several cases have been reported in which, after propranolol, the tachycardia was replaced by a severe bradycardia requiring a demand pacemaker. In one case this resulted after an initial dose of 5 mg propranolol.

IN PATIENTS DURING ANESTHESIA with agents that require catecholamine release for maintenance of adequate cardiac function, beta blockade will impair the desired inotropic effect. Therefore, INDERAL should be titrated carefully when administered for arrhythmias occurring during anesthesia.

IN PATIENTS UNDERGOING MAJOR SURGERY, beta blockade impairs the ability of the heart to respond to reflex stimuli. For this reason, with the exception of pheochromocytoma, INDERAL should be withdrawn 48 hours prior to surgery, at which time all chemical and physiologic effects are gone according to available evidence. However, in case of emergency surgery, since INDERAL is a competitive inhibitor of beta receptor agonists, its effects can be reversed by administration of such agents, e.g., isoproterenol or levarterenol. However, such patients may be subject to protracted severe hypotension. Difficulty in restarting and maintaining the heart beat has also been reported.

IN PATIENTS PRONE TO NONALLERGIC BRONCHOSPASM (e.g., CHRONIC BRONCHITIS, EMPHYSEMA), INDERAL should be administered with caution since it may block bronchodilation produced by endogenous and exogenous catecholamine stimulation of beta receptors.

DIABETICS AND PATIENTS SUBJECT TO HYPOGLYCEMIA: Because of its beta-adrenergic blocking activity, INDERAL may prevent the appearance of premonitory signs and symptoms (pulse rate and pressure changes) of acute hypoglycemia. This is especially important to keep in mind in patients with labile diabetes. Hypoglycemic attacks may be accompanied by a precipitous elevation of blood pressure.

USE IN PREGNANCY: The safe use of INDERAL in human pregnancy has not been established. Use of any drug in pregnancy or women of childbearing potential requires that the possible risk to mother and/or fetus be weighed against the expected therapeutic benefit. Embryotoxic effects have been seen in animal studies at doses about 10 times the maximum recommended human dose.

PRECAUTIONS

Patients receiving catecholamine depleting drugs such as reserpine should be closely observed if INDERAL is administered. The added catecholamine blocking action of this drug may then produce an excessive reduc-

tion of the resting sympathetic nervous activity. Occasionally, the pharmacologic activity of INDERAL may produce hypotension and/or marked bradycardia resulting in vertigo, syncopal attacks, or orthostatic hypotension.

As with any new drug given over prolonged periods, laboratory parameters should be observed at regular intervals. The drug should be used with caution in patients with impaired renal or hepatic function.

ADVERSE REACTIONS

Cardiovascular: bradycardia; congestive heart failure, intensification of AV block; hypotension; paresthesia of hands; arterial insufficiency, usually of the Raynaud type, thrombocytopenic purpura.

Central Nervous System: lightheadedness; mental depression manifested by insomnia, lassitude, weakness, fatigue; reversible mental depression progressing to catatonia; visual disturbances; hallucinations; an acute reversible syndrome characterized by disorientation for time and place, short term memory loss, emotional lability, slightly clouded sensorium, and decreased performance on neuropsychometrics.

Gastrointestinal: nausea, vomiting, epigastric distress, abdominal cramping, diarrhea, constipation, mesenteric arterial thrombosis, ischemic colitis

Allergic: pharyngitis and agranulocytosis, erythematous rash, fever combined with aching and sore throat, laryngospasm and respiratory distress

Respiratory: bronchospasm

Hematologic: agranulocytosis, nonthrombocytopenic purpura, thrombocytopenic purpura

Miscellaneous: reversible alopecia. Oculomucocutaneous reactions involving the skin, serous membranes and conjunctivae reported for a beta blocker (practolol) have not been conclusively associated with propranolol.

Clinical Laboratory Test Findings: Elevated blood urea levels in patients with severe heart disease, elevated serum transaminase, alkaline phosphatase, lactate dehydrogenase

DOSAGE AND ADMINISTRATION
The dosage range for INDERAL is different for each indication.

ORAL

HYPERTENSION—*Dosage must be individualized.*

The usual initial dosage is 40 mg INDERAL twice daily, whether used alone or added to a diuretic. Dosage may be increased gradually until adequate blood pressure is achieved. The usual dosage is 160 to 480 mg per day. In some instances a dosage of 640 mg may be required. The time needed for full hypertensive response to a given dosage is variable and may range from a few days to several weeks.

While twice-daily dosing is effective and can maintain a reduction in blood pressure throughout the day, some patients, especially when lower doses are used, may experience a modest rise in blood pressure toward the end of the 12 hour dosing interval. This can be evaluated by measuring blood pressure near the end of the dosing interval to determine whether satisfactory control is being maintained throughout the day. If control is not adequate, a larger dose, or 3 times daily therapy may achieve better control.

ANGINA PECTORIS—*Dosage must be individualized.*

Starting with 10-20 mg three or four times daily, before meals and at bedtime, dosage should be gradually increased at three to seven day intervals until optimum response is obtained. Although individual patients may respond at any dosage level, the average optimum dosage appears to be 160 mg per day. In angina pectoris, the value and safety of dosage exceeding 320 mg per day have not been established.

If treatment is to be discontinued, reduce dosage gradually over a period of several weeks. (See WARNINGS.)

ARRHYTHMIAS—10-30 mg three or four times daily, before meals and at bedtime.

MIGRAINE—*Dosage must be individualized.*

The initial oral dose is 80 mg INDERAL daily in divided doses. The usual effective dose range is 160-240 mg per day. The dosage may be increased gradually to achieve optimum migraine prophylaxis.

If a satisfactory response is not obtained within four to six weeks after reaching the maximum dose, INDERAL therapy should be discontinued. It may be advisable to withdraw the drug gradually over a period of two weeks.

HYPERTROPHIC SUBAORTIC STENOSIS—20-40 mg three or four times daily, before meals and at bedtime.

PHEOCHROMOCYTOMA—*Preoperatively*—60 mg daily in divided doses for three days prior to surgery, concomitantly with an alpha-adrenergic blocking agent.

—*Management of inoperable tumor*—30 mg daily in divided doses.

PEDIATRIC DOSAGE

At this time the data on the use of the drug in this age group are too limited to permit adequate directions for use.

INTRAVENOUS

Intravenous administration is reserved for life-threatening arrhythmias or those occurring under anesthesia. The usual dose is from 1 to 3 mg administered under careful monitoring, e.g. electrocardiographic, central venous pressure. The rate of administration should not exceed 1 mg (1 ml) per minute to diminish the possibility of lowering blood pressure and causing cardiac standstill. Sufficient time should be allowed for the drug to reach the site of action even when a slow circulation is present. If necessary, a second dose may be given after two minutes. Thereafter, additional drug should not be given in less than four hours. Additional INDERAL should not be given when the desired alteration in rate and/or rhythm is achieved.

Transference to oral therapy should be made as soon as possible.

The intravenous administration of INDERAL has not been evaluated adequately in the management of hypertensive emergencies.

OVERDOSAGE OR EXAGGERATED RESPONSE
IN THE EVENT OF OVERDOSAGE OR EXAGGERATED RESPONSE, THE FOLLOWING MEASURES SHOULD BE EMPLOYED:

BRADYCARDIA—ADMINISTER ATROPINE (0.25 to 1.0 mg): IF THERE IS NO RESPONSE TO VAGAL BLOCKADE, ADMINISTER ISOPROTERENOL CAUTIOUSLY.

CARDIAC FAILURE—DIGITALIZATION AND DIURETICS

HYPOTENSION—VASOPRESSORS, e.g. LEVARTERENOL OR EPINEPHRINE (THERE IS EVIDENCE THAT EPINEPHRINE IS THE DRUG OF CHOICE.)

BRONCHOSPASM—ADMINISTER ISOPROTERENOL AND AMINOPHYLLINE

HOW SUPPLIED
INDERAL
(propranolol hydrochloride)

TABLETS
–Each hexagonal-shaped, orange, scored tablet is embossed with an "I" and imprinted with "INDERAL 10," contains **10 mg** propranolol hydrochloride, in bottles of 100 (NDC 0046-0421-81) and 1,000 (NDC 0046-0421-91). Also in unit dose package of 100 (NDC 0046-0421-99).

–Each hexagonal-shaped, blue, scored tablet is embossed with an "I" and imprinted with "INDERAL 20," contains **20 mg** propranolol hydrochloride, in bottles of 100 (NDC 0046-0422-81) and 1,000 (NDC 0046-0422-91). Also in unit dose package of 100 (NDC 0046-0422-99).

–Each hexagonal-shaped, green, scored tablet is embossed with an "I" and imprinted with "INDERAL 40," contains **40 mg** propranolol hydrochloride, in bottles of 100 (NDC 0046-0424-81) and 1,000 (NDC 0046-0424-91). Also in unit dose package of 100 (NDC 0046-0424-99).

–Each hexagonal-shaped, pink, scored tablet is embossed with an "I" and imprinted with "INDERAL 60," contains **60 mg** propranolol hydrochloride in bottles of 100 (NDC 0046-0426-81) and 1,000 (NDC 0046-0426-91). Also in unit dose package of 100 (NDC 0046-0426-99).

–Each hexagonal-shaped, yellow, scored tablet is embossed with an "I" and imprinted with "INDERAL 80," contains **80 mg** propranolol hydrochloride, in bottles of 100 (NDC 0046-0428-81) and 1,000 (NDC 0046-0428-91). Also in unit dose package of 100 (NDC 0046-0428-99).

The appearance of these tablets is a trademark of Ayerst Laboratories.

Store at room temperature (approximately 25° C).

INJECTABLE
–Each ml contains 1 mg of propranolol hydrochloride in Water for Injection. The pH is adjusted with citric acid. Supplied as: 1 ml ampuls in boxes of 10 (NDC 0046-3265-10).

Store at room temperature (approximately 25° C).

AYERST LABORATORIES INC.
New York, N.Y. 10017

Revised August 1982   241   Printed in U.S.A.

Review Test 1

Suggestions for using this material:

    Go through and write the answers you are sure of.

    Review the word elements and meanings in Lessons 3 through 12.

    Record additional answers that you recall during your review.

    Look up any items remaining and record the answers.

    Check your answers with the key.

    Cover up your answers with a sheet of paper and take the review test again.

Section A

Following are a few of the multitude of terms that are necessary in learning human anatomy. Define each to the extent that you can; some extra words are included to indicate the types of structures described.

1. Celiac artery _____

2. Auricular muscle _____

3. Mastoid process _____

4. Median cubital vein _____

5. Gluteus medius muscle _____

6. Metatarsal arch _____

7. Greater splanchnic nerve _____

8. Dermis _____

9. Plantar surface _____ sole of foot _____

10. Buccinator muscle _____

11. Semispinalis capitis; semispinalis cervicis muscles _____

12. Pectoralis major muscle _____

13. Epithelium (-thel- now is used to refer to any surface) _____

14. Lumbar vertebra _____

15. Inguinal canal _____

16. Olfactory nerve _____

17. Hypophysis; an endocrine gland (formerly pituitary) _____

18. Parotid gland _____

19. Syndesmosis type of joint _____

20. Peroneus muscle _____

21. Intercostal muscles _____

22. Symphysis pubis joint _____

23. Medullary cavity of a bone _____

24. Cerebellar peduncle _____

25. Collateral autonomic ganglion _____

26. Atrioventricular valves of heart _____

27. Tympanic cavity _____

28. Anterior cerebral artery _____

29. Perichondrium _____

30. Synovial membrane _____

31. Aponeurosis of a muscle _____

32. Ischial tuberosity _____

33. Proximal radio-ulnar joint _____

Section B

Analyze the following medical terms by dividing them into their elements. Then give the definition.

1. Anesthetic _____

2. Cephalodynia _____

3. Neurasthenia _____

4. Hyperalgesia _____

5. Carcinogenic ___producing cancer_____

6. Bradycardia ___slow heart_____

7. Phlebectasia ___displacement of vein_____

8. Coronary thrombosis _____

9. Narcolepsy _____

10. Splenorrhagia _____

11. Angioma _____

12. Mitral stenosis _____

13. Pericarditis _____

14. Antiseptic _____

15. Arteriolar _____

16. Myalgia _____

17. Myringotomy _____

18. Ophthalmologist _____

19. Alacrima _____

20. Retinography _____

21. Hematopoiesis _____

22. Hemianopia _____

23. Pelvimetry _____

24. Cardiovascular _____

25. Dyskinesia _____

26. Intracranial _____

27. Hypomenorrhea _____

28. Insomnia _____

29. Cheiloschisis _____

30. Aphasic _____

31. Dipsomania _____

32. Osteolysis _____

33. Tachypnea _____

Section C

Construct terms that fit the following definitions. Words in parentheses are explanatory only.

1. Drooping of internal organs _____

2. Stricture of a vessel _____

3. Instrument to measure the pulse _____

4. Tumor of the meninges _____

5. Swelling (due to accumulation of) lymph _____

6. Softening of the vertebral column _____

7. Rupture of a muscle _____

8. Deficiency of blood _____

9. Pertaining to fever _____

10. Without urine _____

11. Formation of the spleen _____

12. Pertaining to ribs and sternum _____

13. Record of the breast _____

14. Herniation at the navel _____

15. More than normal (number of) digits _____

16. Removal of a nail _____

17. Pertaining to wall of body cavity _____

18. Under the skin _____

19. Fixation of the retina _____

20. Crushing of a vessel _____

21. Pertaining to without life _____

22. Bad (sense of) smell _____

23. Pertaining to thighbone and shinbone _____

24. Instrument to record breathing _____

25. Secrete out _____

26. Inflammation of many arteries _____

27. Pertaining to a large head _____

28. After the removal of a breast _____

29. Pertaining to above the shoulder blade _____

30. Toward the surface _____

31. Pertaining to the back (of the body) _____

32. Pertaining to the middle (of the body) _____

33. Pertaining to the ankle _____

34. Far from _____

35. Flesh-eating _____

36. Across the length _____

37. Incision (to remove a) stone _____

38. Dividing right and left _____

39. Pertaining to a nerve condition _____

Answers to Review Test 1—page 223

Variations on the Theme 2
Sequencing, Plurals, Pronunciation

1. **Sequence of word elements** (sequence, from Latin, meaning to follow)

    As you learn complex terms, you will note that the word elements are used in a particular sequence. Sometimes the sequence is of great importance and a reversal would change the meaning completely. For example:

    hematuria is a condition of blood in the urine

    hemat- = blood, -ur- = urine, -ia = condition

    uremia is a condition of urea in the blood

    -em- = blood, ur- = urea, -ia = condition

    In other terms the sequence is not vital and the order could be reversed without changing the meaning. For example:

    salpingohysterectomy and hysterosalpingectomy both mean removal of the uterus and uterine tubes.

2. **Plurals**

    a. Some of the plural forms of biological terms are the regular English plurals. Other plurals are determined by the Latin or Greek from which they are derived. The following list indicates those that occur frequently in the terminology you are learning.

Singular	Plural	Example
-a	-ae	retina, retinae
-nx	-nges	phalanx, phalanges
-us	-i, -ora	bronchus, bronchi
		corpus, corpora
-is	-es, -ides	testis, testes
		epididymis, epididymides
-x	-ces	cortex, cortices
-um	-a	serum, sera
-on	-a	ganglion, ganglia

    If you are not familiar with the examples used, look them up.

    b. Another problem relating to plurals is whether the plural ending refers to the suffix or to one of the word roots in the term. For example:

    mastectomy = removal of breast (one or two?)

    The plural, mastectomies, would refer to more than one procedure. If both breasts were removed in one procedure the phrase used would be double mastectomy or bilateral mastectomy.

    myeloma = tumor of marrow

    The plural form could be myelomas, myelomata, or, as is usual for this term, multiple myeloma.

3. **Pronunciation** (from Latin, meaning to proclaim)

In this book, pronunciation is given only for the word elements as separate entities. When they are combined, there may be a change in either the sound of a letter or the syllable that is accented. For example:

laryngopharynx	laryngitis
(lar-in-gō-FAR-inks)	(lar-in-JĪ-tis)
thoracotomy	thoracentesis
(thō-ra-KOT-ō-mē)	(tho-ra-sen-TĒ-sis)

It is easy to remember the differences in pronunciation of c and g preceding a vowel. Before e, i, or y, c and g are given their soft pronounciation; before a, o, and u the hard sound is used. (The words gynecology and gynecologist, for which the hard g pronunciation is given preference in the dictionary, represent a notable exception. This preference probably is based on common usage. In most other gyneco- words the soft pronunciation is proper.)

Other helpful tips on pronunciation of consonants include the following:

Ch usually is pronounced like k.	psychology
The p of an initial ps is silent	(sī-KOL-ō-jē)
The initial x is pronounced like z.	xeroderma
	(ze-rō-DER-ma)

Rules for vowel sounds are more complex. Long vowels are marked in this book with a macron (ā); for the subtleties of pronouncing short vowels, see your dictionary.

The primary accent is indicated in this book by capital letters; long words may have one or more secondary accents as well. The primary accent usually is determined as follows:

It is never placed on the last syllable.

It is placed on the next-to-last syllable if the vowel in that syllable is long.

| endocarditis | arteriosclerosis |
| (en-dō-kar-DĪ-tis) | (ar-tē-rē-ō-skle-RŌ-sis) |

If the vowel in the next-to-last syllable is short, the accent is moved back a syllable.

| nephromegaly | gastropathy |
| (nef-rō-MEG-a-lē) | (gas-TROP-a-thē) |

There are many exceptions to these guidelines. Note your instructor's pronunciation and make use of a dictionary.

NOTE: Although you should be on the lookout for the factors of construction mentioned in this lesson, do not be overly concerned about them now. As you use terminology in future courses and in your profession you will become familiar with the variations and eventually you will recognize and use them easily.

TEST YOUR KNOWLEDGE

Give the plurals. Review meanings as you work.

1. Meninx _____

2. Metastasis _____

3. Carpus _____

4. Angioplasty _____

5. Axilla _____

6. Sacrum _____

7. Thorax _____

8. Neurosis _____

9. Costa _____

10. Hematoma _____

11. Plexus _____

12. Cranium _____

13. Medulla _____

14. Appendectomy _____

15. Septum _____

16. Naris _____

17. Alveolus _____

18. Trachea _____

19. Nephron _____

20. Glottis _____

Answers to Lesson 13—page 226

Miscellaneous Word Elements 1

Miscellaneous: from Latin, meaning little mixture

Word Element	Meaning	Aids to Learning	
		Illustrative Words	**Literal Meaning**
adeno- (AD-e-nō)	gland	adenoid	
allo- (AL-ō)	other	allergy	
ambi- (AM-bi)	both	ambidextrous	
-ase (āz)	enzyme		enzyme = in yeast (site of discovery)
-blast	embryonic		germ, bud
caco-, mal- (KAK-ō)	bad	malady, cacophony	
chromo-, chromato- (KRŌ-mō) (krō-MAT-ō)	color	chromosome, Kodachrome, chromium	
-cis- (siz)	cut	excision, scissors	
corpus (KOR-pus)	principal part	incorporate	body
cortico- (KOR-ti-kō)	cortex (outer part)		bark
-cras- (krāz)	mixture	idiosyncrasy	

		Aids to Learning	
Word Element	**Meaning**	**Illustrative Words**	**Literal Meaning**
cyto- (SI-tō)	cell	cytology, cytoplasm	
eti- (Ē-tē)	cause	etiology	
eu- (ū)	good, true	euphonious, euthanasia	
fundus (FUN-dus)	part of organ farthest from exit	profound	base, bottom
-genous (je-nus)	place of origin	endogenous	
-gnosis (NŌ-sis)	knowledge	diagnosis	
histo-, histi- (HIS-tō)	tissue	histiocyte	web
hilus, hilum (HĪ-lus) (HĪ-lum)	attachment point		small thing
-lemma, tunic (LEM-a) (TOO-nik)	covering	neurolemma	sheath
meatus (mē-Ā-tus)	passage	permeate	
-ose (ōs)	carbohydrate, full of	sucrose, verbose	
papilla (pa-PIL-a)	small projection	papilloma	nipple
-philia (FIL-ē-a)	affinity, love	hemophilia, Philadelphia	
-phor-, -fer- (for) (fer)	carry, bear	phosphorus, aquifer	
-phylaxis (fī-LAK-sis)	protection	prophylaxis	guard
plexus (PLEK-sus)	network	complex	braid

	Aids to Learning		
Word Element	Meaning	Illustrative Words	Literal Meaning
pseudo- (SOO-dō)	false	pseudonym	
psychro-, cryo- (SĪ-krō) (KRĪ-ō)	cold	cryogenic	
ramus (RĀ-mus)	branch	ramification	
recto- (REK-tō)	straight	direct, rectify	
reti- (RET-ē)	network	retina	
septum	partition		
-some, somato- (sōm) (sō-MAT-ō)	body	psychosomatic, chromosome	
thermo- (THER-mō)	heat	thermometer	
-ton-, tens- (tōn)	stretch, pull	tense, muscle tone, hypertension	
-top- (tōp)	place	topical medicine, topography	
-trop- (trōp)	turn, influence	gonadotropic	
-troph (trōf)	nourish	atrophy	
tuber (TOO-ber)	swelling, enlargement	tuberculosis	

WORDS USING THESE ELEMENTS

Record words given in class or encountered in your reading.

Word	Meaning

TEST YOUR KNOWLEDGE

Section A

These terms are used in anatomy for parts of organs, etc. Select the proper definition from the list and write it in the blank.

1. Hilum _____Attachment point_____   outer part

2. Tunic _____covering_____   small projection

3. Corpus _____principal part_____   partition

4. Cortex _____outer part_____   network

5. Papilla _____small projection_____   branch

6. Meatus _____passage_____   passage

7. Septum _____partition_____   attachment point

8. Fundus _____part of organ farthest from exit_____   covering

9. Ramus _____branch_____   principal part

10. Plexus _____network_____   part of the organ farthest from exit

Section B

Divide and define the following.

1. Psychrophilic _cold_ ~~mind~~ loving ~~color~~
2. Diagnosis ✓Knowledge through
3. Histology _study of tissue_
4. Peritoneum _stretch around_
5. Adenoid _resembling a gland_
6. Dystrophy _condition of bad nourishment_
7. Eucrasy _condition of good mixture_
8. Chromosome ✓body ~~#~~ color
9. Incision _cut into_
10. Tuberculosis _condition of small swellings_
11. Corticospinal _spinal column cortex_
12. Cryogenic _formation of cold_
13. Anaphylaxis _EXCESSIVE_ ~~without~~ protection
14. Myelogenous _place of origin of marrow_
15. Topical _pertaining to place_

Section C

Construct terms that satisfy the definitions.

1. Instrument to measure heat _thermometer_
2. Affinity for cold _cryophilic_ _psychrophilic_
3. Covering of skeletal muscle _sarcolemma_
4. Without nourishment _Atrophic_ _Atrophy_
5. False pregnancy _pseudocyesis_
6. Pain in a gland _Adenalgia_
7. Making a record with color _chromotography_
8. Deficiency of cells _cytopenia_
9. Nourishing the body _somatotrophic_
10. Study of the cause (of disease) _Etiology_

Section D

Complete the following definitions.

1. Gonad/o/trop/ic *(not troph)* hormone that _influences_ ~~nourishes~~ _____ the reproductive organs

2. Lip/ase _____ _enzyme_ _____ (to digest) fat

3. Tunica media   middle _____ _covering_ _____

4. Oo/phor/on   egg _carry bear_ _____ (ovary)

5. Lateral rectus   muscle _~~branch~~ straight_ _____ on side (of eye)

6. Cyto/lyt/ic   pertaining to destruction of _cells_ _____

7. Iso/ton/ic   pertaining to same _pull_ _____

8. Neuro/hist/o/logy   study of nerve _tissue_ _____

9. Lact/ose   milk _carbohydrate_ _____

10. Top/o/graphy   recording of _place_ _____ (a particular part of the body)

Section E

Complete the following terms.

1. Dia _gnostic_ _____ pertaining to through knowledge

2. Lyso _some_ _____ destructive body

3. Semini _phor fer_ _____ ous pertaining to bearing "seed"

4. Hyper _troph_ _____ y more than normal nourishment (increase in cell size)

5. _____ _cortico_ _____ steroids hormones from the cortex (of the adrenal gland)

6. _____ _eu_ pepsia good digestion

7. _____ _thermo_ gram heat record

8. _____ _chromo_ philic having affinity for color (stain)

9. _____ _pseudo_ esthesic pertaining to false sensation

10. Pro _phylaxis_ _____ protection before (i.e., prevention)

Answers to Lesson 14—page 226

Digestive System

Digestion: from Latin, meaning carry through

To support the chemical processes that maintain life, food, vitamins, minerals, and water must be furnished to each cell constantly. The food that is ingested—carbohydrate, fat, and protein—first requires chemical breakdown. Then it and the other nutrients are absorbed into the blood or lymph to be transported to the cells for use or to a storage area.

The *alimentary canal*, or *digestive tract*, is a 30-foot tube consisting of *oral cavity*, *pharynx*, *esophagus*, *stomach*, *small intestine*, and *large intestine*. Attached to this tube are the *salivary glands*, *liver*, and *pancreas*, which add their secretions to those of the tract, insuring that all enzymes and other necessary materials are present. Bile from the liver accumulates in the *gall bladder* until it is released through a duct to the small intestine. Contraction of muscles in the wall of the tract mixes food with digestive juices and moves material along its length by a wave called *peristalsis*. Rings of muscle called *sphincters* act as valves to control passage from one part to the next. The *peritoneum*, the serous membrane of the abdomen, secretes a fluid that prevents friction during the movements.

		Aids to Learning	
Combining Form	**Anatomical Use**	**Illustrative Words**	**Literal Meaning**
stomato-, oro- (stō-MAT-ō) (Ō-rō)	mouth	oral	
odonto-, dento- (ō-DON-tō) (DEN-tō)	teeth	dentist, orthodontist	
glosso-, linguo- (GLOS-ō) (LING-gwō)	tongue	bilingual, glossolalia	
cheilo-, labio- (KĪ-lō) (LĀ-bē-ō)	lips		
gingivo- (JIN-ji-vō)	gums	gingivitis	
pharyngo- (fa-RING-gō)	pharynx		
palato- (PAL-a-tō)	palate	palatable	

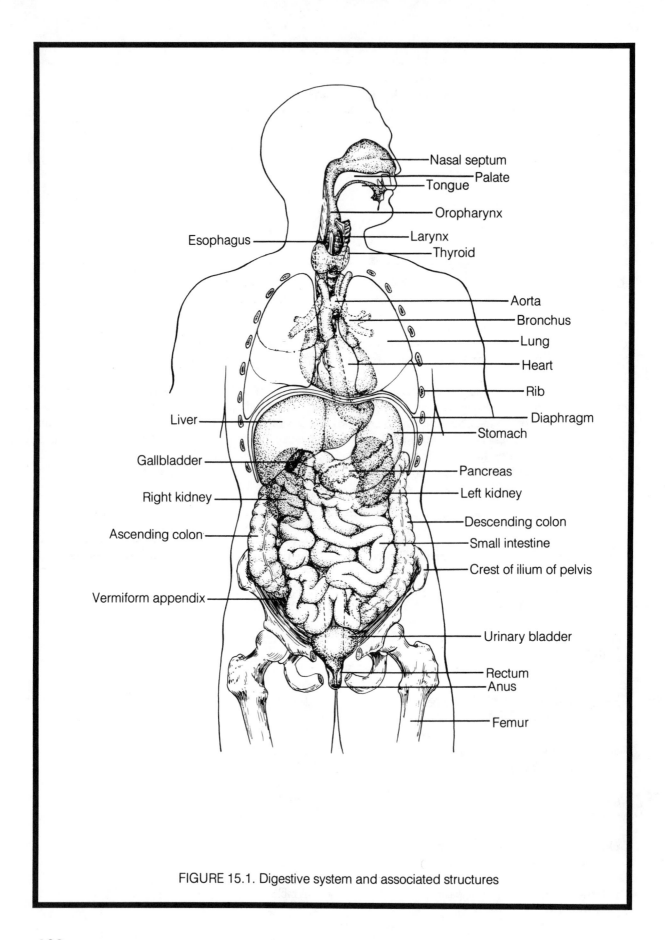

FIGURE 15.1. Digestive system and associated structures

	Aids to Learning		
Combining Form	Anatomical Use	Illustrative Words	Literal Meaning
tonsillo- (TON-sil-ō)	tonsil	tonsillitis	almond (because of shape)
esophago- (ē-SOF-a-gō)	esophagus		carry food
gastro- (GAS-trō)	stomach	gastronomical	
pyloro- (pī-LŌ-rō)	pylorus		gatekeeper
entero- (EN-ter-ō)	intestine	dysentery	
hepato- (HEP-a-tō)	liver	Sal Hepatica	
pancreato- (PAN-krē-a-tō)	pancreas		all flesh
chole-, bili- (KŌ-lē) (BIL-i)	bile, gall	biliary, melancholy	
cysto- (SIS-tō)	bladder		
sphincter (SFINGK-ter)	valve		binder
peritoneo- (per-i-tō-NĒ-ō)	peritoneum	peritonitis	stretch around

Parts of Small Intestine

duodeno- (dū-ō-DĒ-nō)	duodenum	duodenal ulcer	twelve (length in finger-breadths)
jejuno- (je-JOO-nō)	jejunum		empty
ileo- (IL-ē-ō)	ileum	ileostomy	twisted

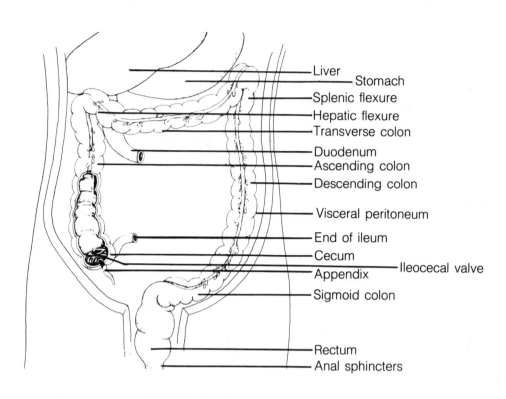

FIGURE 15.2. Large intestine

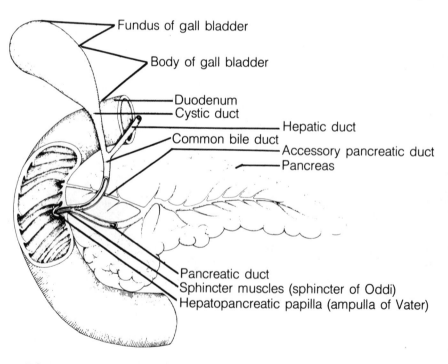

FIGURE 15.3. Pancreas, gall bladder, and duodenum

Parts of Large Intestine			
ceco- (SĒ-kō)	cecum		blind
appendico- (a-PEN-di-kō)	appendix	appendectomy	hang to
colo- (KŌ-lō)	colon	colitis	shorten
recto- (REK-tō)	rectum		straight
procto- (PROK-tō)	rectum and anus	proctologist	
ano- (A-nō)	anus		anus = ring

WORDS USING THESE ELEMENTS

Record words given in class or encountered in your reading.

Word	Meaning

TEST YOUR KNOWLEDGE

Section A

What part of the digestive system is referred to by each of the following?

1. Gastro- _____ stomach _____
2. Colo- _____ colon _____
3. Hepato- _____ liver _____
4. Procto- _____ rectum & anus _____
5. Pancreato- _____ pancreas _____
6. Glosso- _____ tongue _____
7. Entero- _____ intestine _____
8. Esophago- _____ esophagus _____
9. Pharyngo- _____ pharnyx _____
10. Stomato- _____ mouth _____

Section B

Divide and define the following terms.

1. Palatoschisis _____ splitting of palates _____ palates
2. Pyloric sphincter _____ pertaining to pylorus valve _____
3. Duodenal _____ pertaining to duodenum _____
4. Tonsillectomy _____ removal of tonsil _____
5. Cheilorrhaphy (see Lesson 16) _____ suture in lip _____
6. Pharyngotympanic _____ pertaining to membrane of the pharynx & ear _____
7. Gastroplegia _____ paralysis of the stomach _____
8. Dysentery _____ painful intestine. _____
9. Peritonitis _____ inflammation stretching around of peritoneum _____
10. Cholelithotripsy _____ crushing gall stone _____
11. Odontoid _____ resembling teeth _____
12. Stomatoma _____ tumor in the mouth _____
13. Oropharynx _____ mouth _____
14. Sphincteralgia _____ pain in valve _____
15. Exodontia _____ condition of _____ removal of a tooth _____

Section C

Construct terms for the following.

1. Pertaining to tongue and pharynx ___glossopharyngEAl___
2. Specialist in rectum and anus ___proctologist___
3. Herniation of the stomach ___gAstrocEle___ _cele_
4. Pertaining to ileum and cecum ___ileocecAl___
5. Examination of the colon ___coloscopy___
6. Inflammation of the gums ___gingivitis___
7. Disease of the teeth ___~~orthopathy~~___ ___odontopathy___
8. Pain in stomach and rectum ___proctAlgiA___ ___gAstrorectAlgiA___
9. Enlargement of the liver ___hEpAtomEgAly___
10. Originating in the pancreas ___pAncrEAtogEnous___   _gnosis_ _genous_

Section D

Complete the following definitions.

1. Denti/lingu/al   pertaining to ___tEEth___ and ___tongue___
2. Tonsill/o/lith   stone in a ___tonsil___
3. Chol/emic   pertaining to ___bilE___ in the blood
4. Appendic/o/stomy   new opening from the ___AppEndix___
5. Per/or/al   through the ___mouth___
6. Proct/o/stenosis   stricture of the ___rEctum & Anus___
7. Bili/rubin   pigment of the ___bilE___
8. Enter/o/sepsis   infection in the ___intEstinE___
9. Hepatic/o/lith/iasis   stone in the ___livEr___ duct
10. Pharyng/o/rhin/itis   inflammation of the naso- ___pharnyx___

Section E

Complete the following terms.

1. ___chEilo___ phagia   eating (biting) the lips
2. ___rEcto___ pexy   fixation of the rectum
3. ___gAstro___ rrhea   flow (of secretion) in the stomach
4. ___~~bilE cysto~~___ / ___cholEcysto___ kinin   hormone that moves the gall bladder (causes contraction)

113

5. Extra _peritoneal_____   outside of the peritoneum

6. _____ _ileocec_____al   pertaining to ileum and cecum

7. _____ _colo_ ptosis   drooping of the colon

8. _____ _esophago_ cele   herniation of the esophagus

9. _____ _stomato_ dysodia   bad odor from the mouth

10. Hypo _glossal_____   under the tongue

Answers to Lesson 15—page 228

Following are diagrams of the digestive system. On each label line, write in the name of the part.

Write each term or combining form on the appropriate label line.

Ano-
Appendico-
Cheilo-, labio-
Cholecysto-
Colo-
Entero-
Esophago-
Gastro-
Glosso-, linguo-
Hepato-
Oropharynx
Palato-
Pancreato-
Recto-

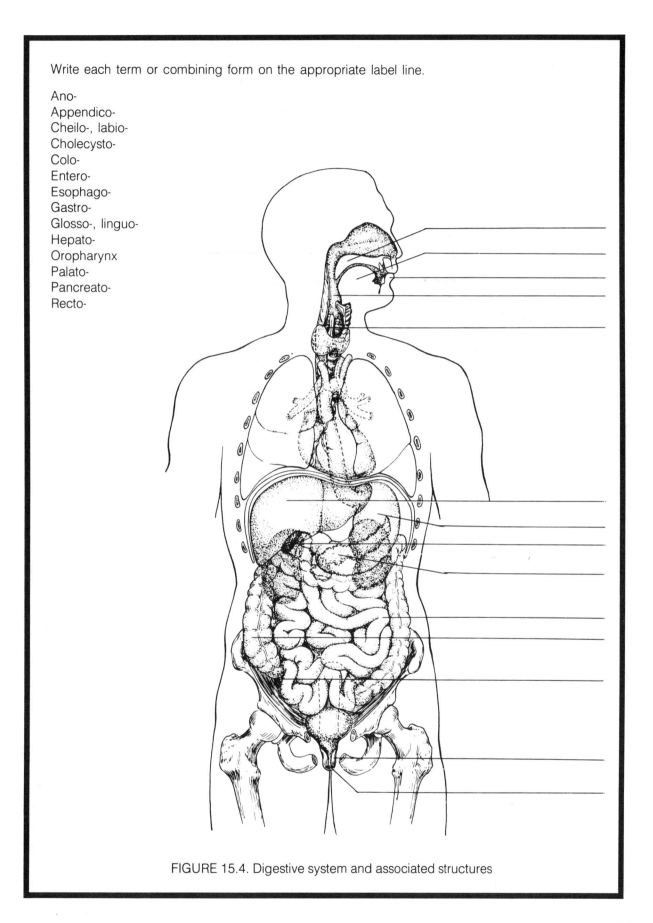

FIGURE 15.4. Digestive system and associated structures

Write each term or combining form on the appropriate label line.

Anal
Appendico-
Ceco-
Colo-
Duodeno-
Gastro-
Hepato-
Ileo-
Ileocecal
Recto-
Transverse
Visceral peritoneum

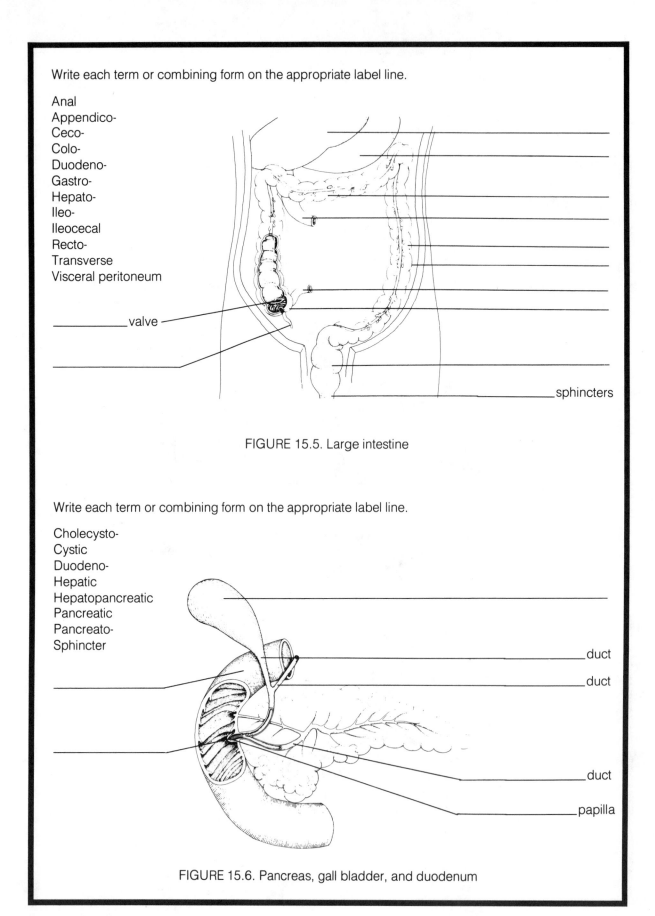

_____ valve

_____ sphincters

FIGURE 15.5. Large intestine

Write each term or combining form on the appropriate label line.

Cholecysto-
Cystic
Duodeno-
Hepatic
Hepatopancreatic
Pancreatic
Pancreato-
Sphincter

_____ duct

_____ duct

_____ duct

_____ papilla

FIGURE 15.6. Pancreas, gall bladder, and duodenum

116

CROSSWORD 1

Digestive System

This crossword puzzle is reprinted from a book of word puzzles for health professionals. Some of the answers are in this lesson, some you can find in the Index or in Appendix B and some are common knowledge. Fill in as many answers as you can. By checking your answers you also will learn some terms that are not in this book.

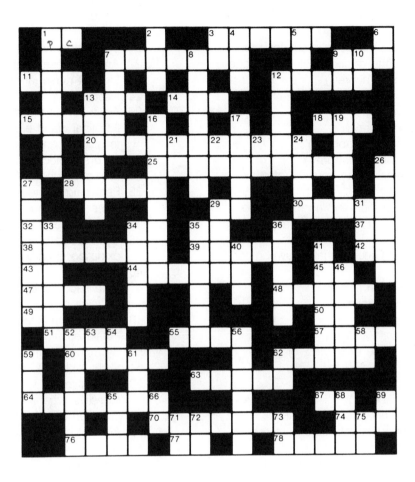

Solution is on page 229.

Across

1. After meals (Latin abbrev.)
3. Queasiness or unpleasant sensation; often referred to the abdomen; frequently results in vomiting
7. Movement of solvent across a semipermeable membrane from lesser to greater concentration
9. Bowel or intestine
11. Review of systems (abbrev.)
12. Tenth cranial nerve; innervates muscles of pharynx, larynx, esophagus, thoracic and abdominal viscera, pancreas, and gastric glands

Down

1. An organic nitrogenous compound formed by combinations of amino acids and their derivatives
2. Basal metabolic rate (abbrev.)
3. Nickel (symbol)
4. Request
5. Equal Rights Amendment (abbrev.)
6. Physical therapy (abbrev.)
7. Excessively fat
8. Characterized by spasms
9. Genitourinary (abbrev.)
10. We
12. Regurgitate

Across

13. According to
14. Retch; attempt to vomit
15. Excrement discharged from intestine
18. Hydrochloric acid (symbol)
20. Wave of contraction by which alimentary canal propels its contents
25. Referring to or caused by food or nourishment
28. Largest organ in the body; produces bile, converts sugars to glycogen, stores glycogen
29. Bowel movement (abbrev.)
30. Liquid introduced into the rectum
32. Chromium (symbol)
34. Mental health (abbrev.)
35. Myocardial infarction (abbrev.)
37. Occupational therapy (abbrev.)
38. That which remains after removal of other substances; roughage
39. Gradual disintegration and necrosis of the tissue due to loss of substance on a mucous surface
42. Twelfth letter of Greek alphabet; symbol for micron
43. Before meals (Latin abbrev.)
44. Carcinoma and sarcoma
45. Aluminum (symbol)
47. Immediately (Latin abbrev.)
48. Mass of food to be swallowed, or a mass moving along the intestines
49. Each (abbrev.)
50. Intramuscular (abbrev.)
51. Fleshy folds at orifice of the mouth
55. Bladder; reservoir for bile on the inferior surface of the liver
57. Vessel that conveys blood toward or to the heart
60. Growth elevated above the surface of the mucosa and extending into the lumen of a body cavity
62. Mild or soothing type diet
63. Any of a group of fats or fat-like substances that are insoluble in water, including true fats, lipoids, sterols, and hydrocarbons
64. Milk sugar
67. Orifice; mouth
70. Proteolytic enzyme of pancreatic secretion
74. American Gastroenterological Association (abbrev.)
76. Masticate
77. *Nursing Research* (abbrev.)
78. Prefix indicating sweetness

Down

13. Gastric enzyme; breaks peptide linkages, changing proteins into proteoses and peptones
16. Abnormal liquidity and frequency of feces
17. Portion of small intestine between jejunum and cecum
19. Mixture of partially digested food, saliva, and gastric juice
21. Slight (abbrev.)
22. Ante meridiem (abbrev.)
23. Student nurse (abbrev.)
24. Keep; safeguard
26. Air or gas in the stomach or intestine
27. Intestinal gland enzyme that converts sucrose to glucose and fructose
29. Fluid secreted by the liver
31. Milk of magnesia (abbrev.)
33. Pertaining to the rectum
34. Slime of the mucous membranes
35. Mucous membrane
36. Cycle constituting final common pathway in oxidation of carbohydrate, fat, and protein
40. Sob
41. Fluid secreted by the salivary glands, contains ptyalin
46. Cavity within a tubular organ
52. Potent emetic
53. By mouth (Latin abbrev.)
54. Slight (abbrev.)
56. Fat splitting or lipolytic enzyme found in digestive organs and blood
58. Freudian term for the true unconscious
59. Amount of heat required to raise 1 g of water 1° C (abbrev.)
61. Affirmative
62. Birthday (abbrev.)
65. Single thing
66. Enterostomal therapist (abbrev.)
68. Pouch
69. Double-lumen tube used for intestinal decompression (abbrev.)
71. Registered nurse (abbrev.)
72. Year (abbrev.)
73. Nasogastric (abbrev.)
75. Proceed

TERMINOLOGY SEARCH 3: PATIENT DISCHARGE SUMMARY

A patient discharge summary contains a number of terms and abbreviations with which you should now be familiar. This one—anonymous, of course (from Greek, meaning without a name)—is a good example.

DISCHARGE SUMMARY

PATIENTS NAME: **MEDICAL RECORD NO:**
(Last-First-MI)

ADMITTED: **DISCHARGED:**   **SERVICE:**

ADMITTING DIAGNOSIS: 1.   Rest pain of left foot.

DISCHARGE DIAGNOSIS: 1.   Atherosclerotic peripheral vascular disease.

ATTENDING: Dr. A

PROCEDURE: 1.   Aortofemoral angiogram.
              2.   Left femoral posterior tibial graft reverse saphenous vein
              3.   Left superficial femoral artery endarterectomy
              4.   Two intraoperative arteriograms

DATE OF PROCEDURES: 2-20-84

HISTORY OF PRESENT ILLNESS: This 78-year-old black male was recently admitted to the Medical College of Virginia with a two-month history of progressive rest pain of toes of left foot. Angiogram at that time revealed stenotic lesion of left profunda and no distal bypassable vessels. Only the left posterior tibial was opacified. Dopplers revealed adequate flow to the ankle but no signals at toes. The patient underwent left profundoplasty and was discharged on 2-02-84. Since discharge, he has had severe rest pain in the left toes which keeps him awake at night and was not relieved by pain medications. Over the week preceding admission, he noted cyanosis, cooling and tissue breakdown of the left second and third toes

PAST MEDICAL HISTORY: Significant for surgeries as per History of Present Illness. History of peptic ulcer disease. No known allergies. Current medications are Percocet and Colace.

SOCIAL HISTORY: He is an occasional smoker over the last 40 years. Ethanol — negative.

REVIEW OF SYSTEMS: Negative.

PHYSICAL EXAMINATION: This is an elderly black male in no acute distress. HEENT: Remarkable for arcus senilis and muddy sclerae. Neck: Supple with jugulovenous distention at 45 degrees. Carotids 2 + with palpable thrill on the right. Bilateral bruit with right greater than left. Chest: Clear. Heart: Regular rate and rhythm with Grade III/VI systolic ejection murmur at the left lower sternal border. Abdomen: Scaphoid and soft. Positive bowel sounds. GU: Normal. Uncircumcised male. Rectal: 4 + enlarged prostate. Heme negative. Extremities: Positive arthritic changes of both hands.

PATIENT'S NAME:
(Last-First-MI)

There is muscle wasting of the left lower extemity. The left foot was cooler than the right. There was capillary refill which was delayed on the left as compared to the right. Pulses in the left extremity were only by Doppler. There was 1 + dorsalis pedis on the right.

LABORATORY DATA: Initial laboratory remarkable for hemoglobin of 9.8, white blood cell count 6.3. The patient was admitted and had an aortofemoral angiogram remarkable for superficial femoral artery being occluded in distal thigh and only the posterior tibial artery opacified in the leg.

HOSPITAL COURSE: The patient was admitted and underwent the above angiogram. It was felt to be unchanged from previous angiogram. The patient was preoped and taken to the Operating Room on 2-20-84 after receiving two units of blood for low hemoglobin. He had a left distal superficial femoral artery to posterior tibial artery bypass graft using a reverse saphenous vein. In addition, he underwent left superficial femoral endarterectomy and two intraoperative arteriograms. The procedures were performed by Dr. A with assistance by Dr. B and Dr. C. The patient tolerated the procedure well. Post-operative ankle arm ratios on the left were .53 as compared to preoperative ankle arm ratios of .3. Ankle arm index improved on the second post-operative day to .53. The patient was evaluated by Urology for difficulty voiding and enlarged prostate and recommended transurethral resection of the prostate. Post-operatively, his ankle arm pressures had risen to 86/120 as compared to preoperatively only 60/140. The patient had continued to complain of some left foot pain although the foot was noticeably warmer than preoperatively. Physical Therapy saw the patient throughout his postoperative course. He was gradually ambulated. He once again had two units of blood transfused for low hemoglobin. Because of history of forty pound weight loss, the patient had barium enema and upper G.I. which were all normal. He had a CA drawn which returned 3.7 and his acid phosphatase times two was .6. The patient at the time of discharge was able to ambulate reasonably well with a cane.

FOLLOW-UP: The patient will return to see Dr. A in his office in six weeks and return to see Dr. B in his office in two weeks. He is to take aspirin 1 tablet qam, Persantine 1 tab t.i.d.

D: 3-07-84   Dr. A, M.D.
T: 3-10-84
(2769)

VIRGINIA COMMONWEALTH UNIVERSITY
Medical College of Virginia Hospitals
Richmond, Virginia 23298

FORM A-464 MR-20 (6-1-76)
OPI: Department of Medical Records

cards – ✓

Medical Procedures

Procedure: from Latin, meaning go forward

This lesson presents a few of the most commonly used terms for medical procedures. You already will be familiar with many of them. Some of them (e.g., centesis, ostomy, therapy, and stasis) also are used as separate words.

		Aids to Learning	
Word Element	**Meaning**	**Illustrative Words**	**Literal Meaning**
-centesis (sen-TĒ-sis)	puncture	amniocentesis	
-clysis (KLĪ-sis)	irrigation		drenching
-ectomy (EK-tō-mē)	removal	tonsillectomy	cut out
-graphy (GRAF-ē)	recording	cardiography, stenography	write
-iatrist (Ī-a-trist)	healer	podiatrist	
-iatry (Ī-a-trē)	healing	psychiatry	
-pexy (PEK-sē)	fixation		
-plasty (PLAS-tē)	repair, plastic surgery	dermatoplasty	form
prostho- (PROS-thō)	addition	prosthesis	put to
-rrhaphy (RA-fē)	suture		
-scopy (SKŌ-pē)	examination	microscopy	

	Aids to Learning		
Word Element	Meaning	Illustrative Words	Literal Meaning
-stasis (STĀ-sis)	stopping, standing still	homeostasis, hemostasis	
-stomy, -ostomy (STŌ-mē) (OS-tō-mē)	formation of new opening	colostomy	mouth
-therapy (THER-a-pē)	treatment	chemotherapy	
-tomy (TŌ-mē)	incision	tracheotomy	cut
-tripsy (TRIP-sē)	crushing		rubbing

WORDS USING THESE ELEMENTS

Record words given in class or encountered in your reading.

Word	Meaning
_____	_____
_____	_____
_____	_____
_____	_____
_____	_____
_____	_____
_____	_____
_____	_____
_____	_____
_____	_____
_____	_____

TEST YOUR KNOWLEDGE

Section A

Divide and define the following terms.

1. Colostomy _formation of a new opening in the colon_
2. Thoracocentesis _puncture the thorax_
3. Splenopexy _fixation of the spleen_
4. Hemostasis _stopping blood_
5. Psychotherapy _treatment of the mind_
6. Omphalotripsy _crushing friction on the umbilicus_
7. Keratoplasty _repair of the cornea_
8. Cardiography _recording of the heart_
9. Pediatry _healing of children_
10. Gastroclysis _irrigation of the stomach_
11. Pancreatopexy _fixation of the pancreas_
12. Laparotomy _incision into the abdominal wall_
13. Cheilorrhaphy _suture in the lip_
14. Hepatocentesis _puncture the liver_
15. Psychiatrist _specialist in the ~~study~~ healer of the mind_
16. Ileostomy _formation of a new ~~hole~~ opening in the ileum_
17. Tracheotomy (see Lesson 17) _incision in the trachea_
18. Angiotripsy _crushing friction on a vessel_
19. Prosthodontics _pertaining to addition of teeth_
20. Cholestasis _stopping bile_

Section B

Construct terms for the following phrases.

1. Removal of the spleen _splenectomy_
2. Incision into the pancreas _pancreatotomy_
3. Repair of the nose _nasoplasty_ _rhinoplasty_
4. Recording of the brain _graphy_ _encephalogram_
5. Examination of a joint _articuloscope_ _arthroscopy_
6. Treatment (with) water _aqueoustherapy_ _hydrotherapy_
7. Puncture of a vein _venocentesis_

123

8. Formation of new opening from the trachea _tracheostomy_

9. Irrigation of the mouth _stomatoclysis / orochysis_

10. Suture of the palate _palatorrhaphy_

Section C

Complete the following definitions.

1. Pod/iatry _~~study of~~ healing_ of the feet

2. Prosthet/ic   pertaining to an _addition_

3. Col/o/lysis _destruction_ of the colon

4. Phren/o/pexy _fixation_ of the diaphragm

5. Therapeut/ic   pertaining to _treatment_

6. Chole/stasis _stopping_ (flow) of bile

7. Muco/stat/ic   pertaining to _stopping_ (flow) of mucus

8. Vas/ectomy _removal_ of (a portion of) the vas deferens

9. Nephr/o/tomy _incision_ into the kidney

10. Pyel/o/graphy _recording_ of the kidney pelvis

Section D

Complete the following terms.

1. Amnio _centesis_   puncture of the amnion

2. Homeo _stasis_   standing the same

3. Cysto _graphy_   recording of the bladder

4. Colpo _rrhaphy_   suturing of the vagina

5. Oto _scope_   pertaining to examination of the ear

6. Thoraco _tomy_   incision into the thorax

7. Hyster _ectomy_   removal of the uterus

8. Hemiphalang _ectomy_   removal of half of a digit bone

9. Ureteroprocto _stomy_   formation of a new opening between ureter and rectum

10. Dermato _plasty_   plastic surgery on the skin

Answers to Lesson 16—page 229

Respiratory and Endocrine Systems

> **Respiratory:** from Latin, meaning breathe back
> **Endocrine:** from Greek, meaning separate within

The basic process that releases the energy that maintains life can be expressed in its simplest form as:

food + oxygen ⟶ carbon dioxide + water + energy

The exchange of gases with the environment is essential, since there must be a constant flow of oxygen to the cells and a constant flow of carbon dioxide away from them. This vital exchange, the function of the respiratory system, occurs in the *lungs*, where bood in the *pulmonary* capillaries is exposed to air in *alveoli*. The surface area involved in this exchange is approximately equivalent to the area of a tennis court. The *nasal cavity, pharynx, larynx, trachea*, and a many-branched *bronchial* "tree" carry air to and from the alveoli. Breathing occurs when muscles, *diaphragm*, and *intercostals* alternately contract and relax, changing pressure in the thoracic cavity and thus causing inflation and deflation of the lungs. Friction is prevented by the fluid secretion of the *pleura*, the serous membrane associated with these organs.

The endocrine system is the only system of the body in which the organs are not structurally connected. It consists of a number of glands that secrete their hormones directly into the blood. These hormones exert their effects on specific "target tissue" to maintain the complex chemical balance referred to as *homeostasis*. There is much interaction between hormones, and appropriate levels are preserved by means of feedback loops. The *hypothalamus* of the brain also plays an important role in regulating the secretion of hormones by these glands. The major endocrine glands are the *thyroid, parathyroids, pancreas, adrenal, ovaries, testes*, and *hypophysis* (pituitary).

	Aids to Learning		
Combining Form	**Anatomical Use**	**Common Name**	**Literal Meaning**
Respiratory System			
naris (NĀ-ris)	nostril		
naso-, rhino- (NĀ-zō) (RĪ-nō)	nose		
sino-, sinus (SĪ-nō) (SĪ-nus)	sinus		a hollow
pharyngo- (fa-RING-gō)	pharynx	throat	
laryngo- (la-RING-gō)	larynx	voice box	
glott-	glottis	opening to larynx	back of tongue

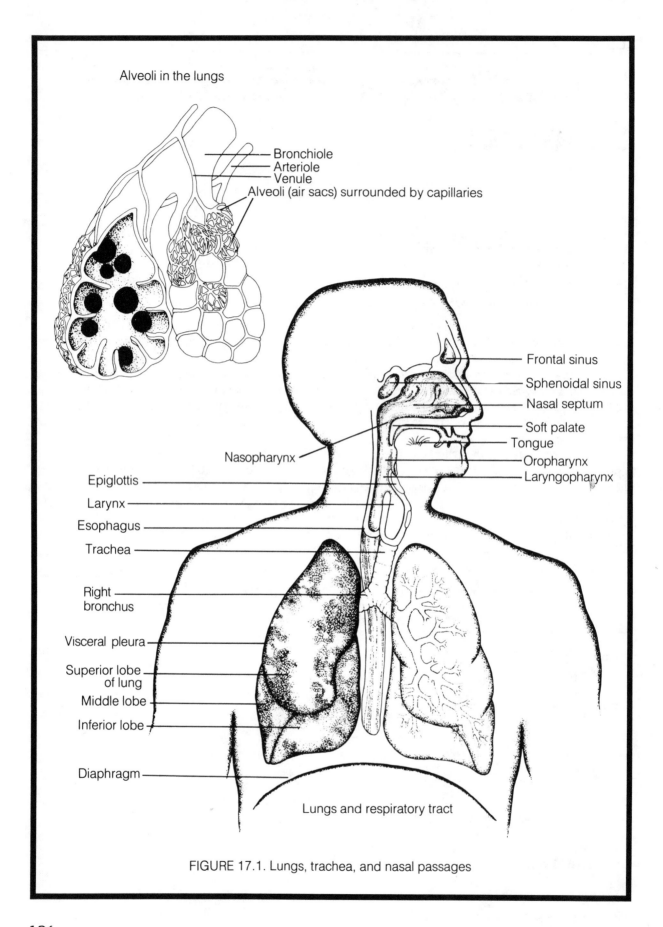

Alveoli in the lungs

Bronchiole
Arteriole
Venule
Alveoli (air sacs) surrounded by capillaries

Frontal sinus
Sphenoidal sinus
Nasal septum
Soft palate
Tongue
Oropharynx
Laryngopharynx

Nasopharynx

Epiglottis
Larynx
Esophagus
Trachea

Right bronchus

Visceral pleura
Superior lobe of lung
Middle lobe
Inferior lobe

Diaphragm

Lungs and respiratory tract

FIGURE 17.1. Lungs, trachea, and nasal passages

Combining Form	Anatomical Use	Common Name	Literal Meaning
tracheo- (TRĀ-kē-ō)	trachea	windpipe	rough (due to cartilage)
broncho-, bronchi- (BRONG-kō) (BRONG-kē)	bronchus	bronchial tube	
pneumo-, pneumono- (NŪ-mō) (nū-MŌ-nō)	lung		
pulmo-, pulmono- (PUL-mō) (PUL-mō-nō)			
pleuro- (PLOO-rō)	pleura	membrane of lungs	side
alveolo- (al-VĒ-ō-lō)	alveolus	microscopic air space of lung	little cavity
phreno- (FREN-ō)	diaphragm		diaphragm = fence across

Endocrine System

Combining Form	Anatomical Use	Common Name	Literal Meaning
hypophyseo-, pituit- (hī-POF-iz-ē-ō) (pi-TŪ-it)	hypophysis	pituitary gland	hypophysis = grow under; pituit = phlegm (thick mucus)
adreno-, suprareno- (a-DRĒ-nō) (soo-pra-RĒ-nō)	suprarenal	adrenal gland	adrenal = toward kidney; suprarenal = above kidney
thyro- (THĪ-rō)	thyroid		resembling a shield
parathyro- (par-a-THĪ-rō)	parathyroid		beside thyroid
pancreato- (PAN-krē-at-ō)	pancreas		all flesh
oophoro-, ovario- (ō-OF-ō-rō) (ō-VĀ-rē-ō)	ovary		oophor = egg-bearer
orchido-, testi- (OR-ki-dō) (TES-ti)	testis		testi = witness

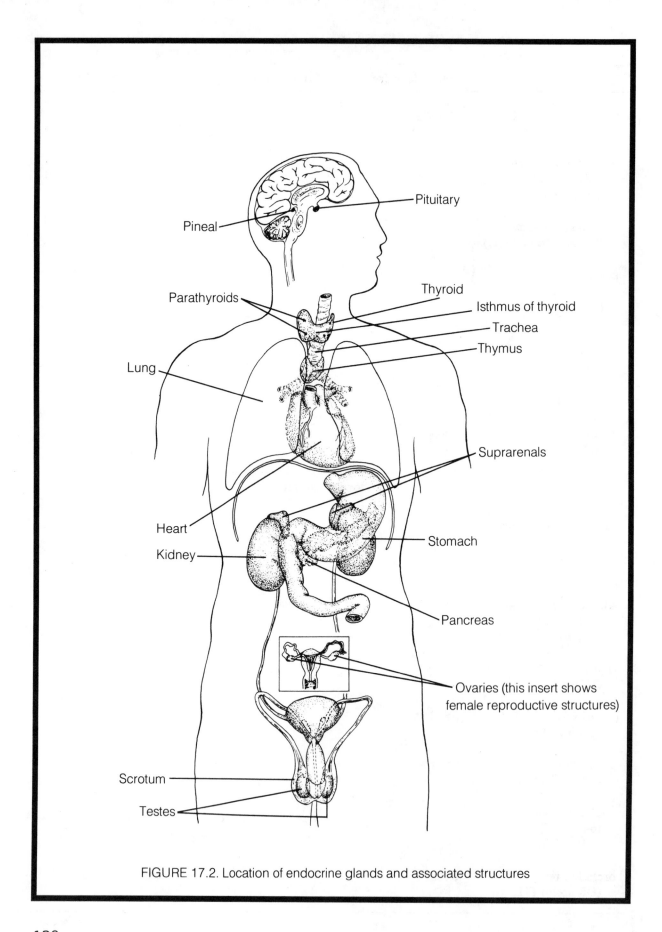

FIGURE 17.2. Location of endocrine glands and associated structures

WORDS USING THESE ELEMENTS

Record words given in class or encountered in your reading.

Word	Meaning

TEST YOUR KNOWLEDGE

Section A

Divide and define the following terms.

1. Hypophysectomy _removal of hypophysis_
2. Thyroadenitis _inflammation of thyroid gland_
3. Epiglottis _above upon the glottis_
4. Pulmonary _pertaining to the lung_
5. Pleuroscopy _examination of the ~~lungs~~ pleura_
6. Phrenoptosis _drooping of the diaphram_
7. Pancreatolith _stone in pancreas_
8. Rhinorrhagia _extreme flow from nose_
9. Nasolacrimal _pertaining to tears and nose_
10. Laryngoplegia _paralysis of the larynx_
11. Pneumonectomy _removal of lung_
12. Phrenospasm _spasm of the diaphram_
13. Sinusitis _inflammation of sinus_

14. Bronchiectasis   _dilitation of bronchus_

15. Laryngocele   _herniation of the larynx_

16. Alveolar   _pertaining to the aveolus_

17. Adrenotropic   _suprarenal_

18. Pleurisy (from pleuritis)   _condition of inflammed plurea_

19. Tracheoplasty   _repair of the trachea_

20. Bronchopneumonia   _____

Section B

Construct terms for the following definitions.

1. Enlargement of the thyroid   _megaly_

2. Tumor of the pancreas   _pancreatoma_

3. Puncture of the ovary   _oophoro centecis_

4. Examination of the bronchus   _broncho scopy_

5. Instrument to examine the larynx   _laryngo scope_

6. Pain in the pleura   _pleur algia_

7. Abnormal condition of the lungs   _pulmonosis_

8. Record of a sinus   _sinu graph_

9. Disease of the pancreas   _pancreato_

10. Removal of the larynx   _laryngeal ectopy_

Section C

Complete the following definitions.

1. External nares   external _nostrils_

2. Pleur/o/pneumon/ia   condition of _lung_ and _pleura_

3. Parathyroid/oma   tumor of the _parathyroid_

4. Pneum/o/melan/osis   black conditon of the _lung_

5. Peri/pharyng/eal   pertaining to around the _pharynx_

6. Endo/trach/eal   pertaining to within the _trachea_

7. Ovari/o/pathy   disease of the _ovary_

8. Orchid/oncus   tumor of the _testis_

9. Phren/algia   pain in the _diaphram_

10. Sinus/oid   resembling a _sinus_

130

Section D

Complete the following terms.

1. Hypo_____*pituit*_____ism — less than normal (activity) of the pituitary

2. _____*bronchoaveol*_____ itis — inflammation of alveoli and bronchioles

3. _____*Adeno*_____ tropin — (hormone) to influence the adrenal cortex

4. Hyper _____*thyroid*_____ — more than normal (activity) of the thyroid

5. _____*strepto*_____ cocci — spherical (bacteria infecting) the lung

6. _____*pharngia*_____ xerosis — dryness of the pharynx

7. _____*trachea*_____ malacia — softening of (cartilage) of the trachea

8. Crypt_____*orchid*_____ism — hidden testis

9. _____*phreno*_____ tripsy — crushing of the (nerve to) the diaphragm

10. _____*nasal*_____ septum — septum of the nose
    _____*narl*_____

Answers to Lesson 17—page 231

Following are diagrams of the respiratory and endocrine systems. On each label line, write in the name of the part.

131

Write each term or combining form on the appropriate label line.

Alveolo-
Broncho-, bronchi-
Epiglottis
Inferior
Laryngo-
Laryngopharynx

Naris
Nasal
Nasopharynx
Oropharynx
Phreno-
Pneumo-, pneumono-, pulmo-, pulmono-

Sino-, sinus-
Superior
Tracheo-
Visceral pleura

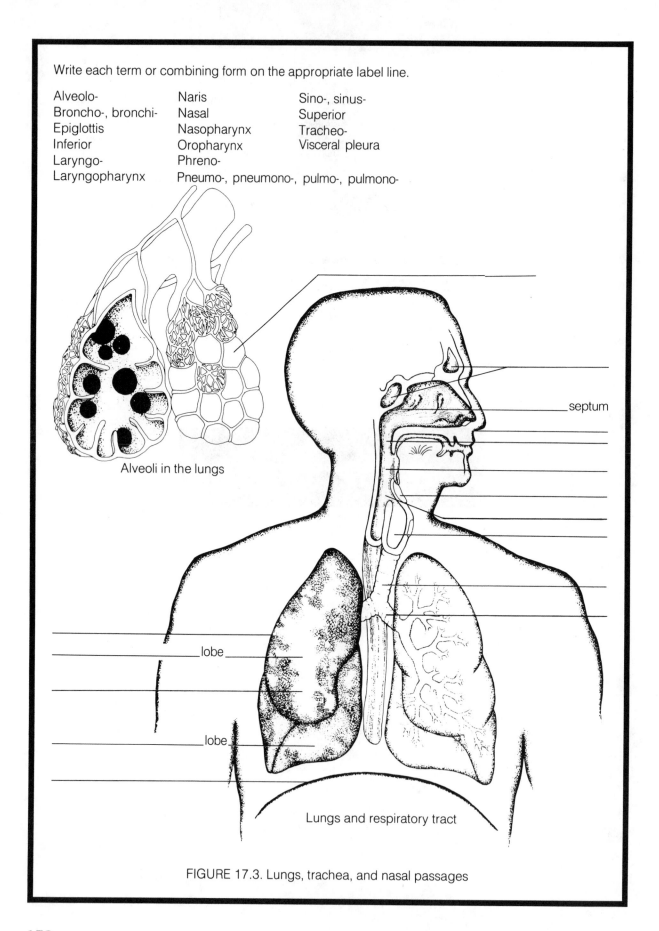

Alveoli in the lungs

septum

lobe

lobe

Lungs and respiratory tract

FIGURE 17.3. Lungs, trachea, and nasal passages

Write each combining form on the appropriate label line.

Adreno-, suprareno-
Hypophyseo-, pituit-
Orchido-, testi-
Oophoro-, ovario-
Pancreato-
Parathyro-
Thyro-

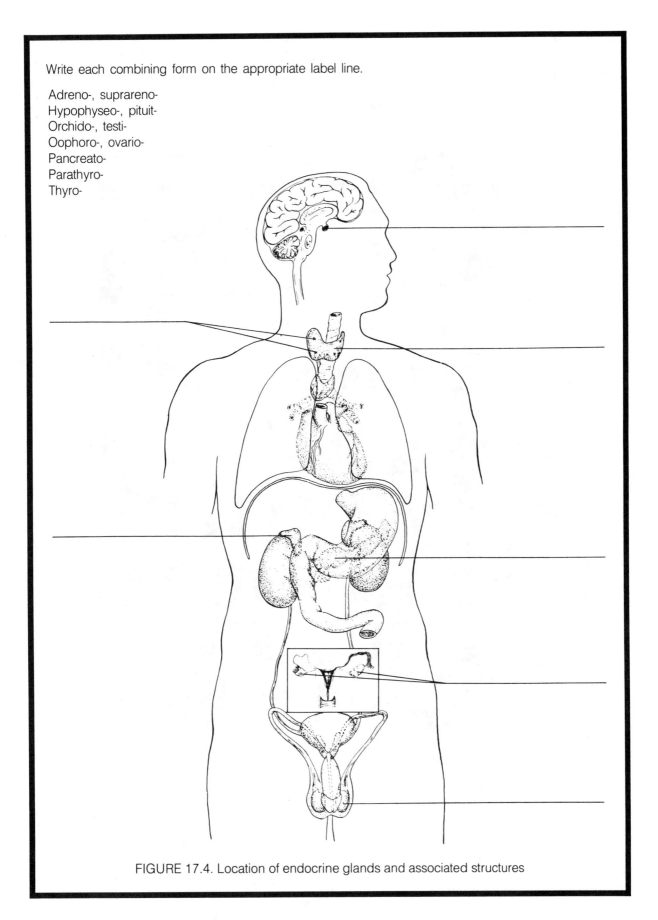

FIGURE 17.4. Location of endocrine glands and associated structures

CROSSWORD 2

Respiration

This crossword puzzle is reprinted from a book of word puzzles for health professionals. Some of the answers are in this lesson, some you can find in the Index or in Appendix B, and some are common knowledge. Fill in as many answers as you can. By checking your answers you also will learn some terms that are not in this book.

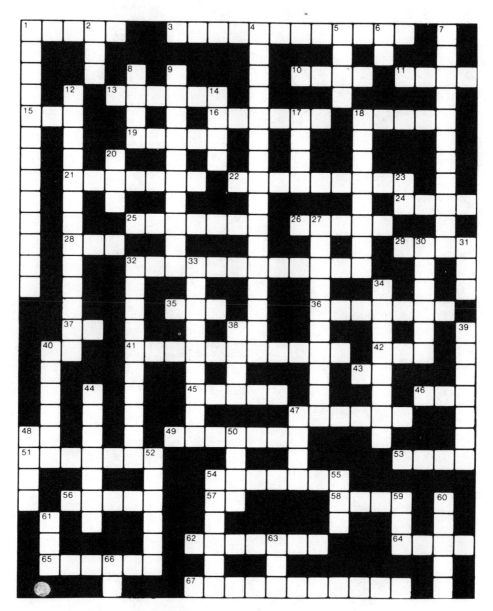

Solution is on page 232.

Across

1. Expectorate secretions from the lungs
3. Surgically created airway
10. Large anatomical division of the lungs
11. Number of breaths per minute
13. Separates the nares
15. Mono-

Down

1. Gas given off with expiration (two words)
2. CO_2 or O_2
4. Increase in rate or depth of respiration leading to loss of carbon dioxide
5. Metal or plastic device placed in a tracheostomy

Across

16. Natural or artificial passage necessary for breathing
18. Thorax
19. Nostrils
21. Use of vacuum to clear an airway
22. Infectious disease of the lungs; formerly #1 cause of death
24. Cyanosis is first seen in the _____ bed
25. Divisions of the trachea leading to each lung
26. Quality of stertorous breathing
28. Number of lungs normally possessed by humans
29. Not shallow
32. Act of breathing (pl.)
35. Influenza (colloq.)
36. State of oxygen deficiency
37. Oxygen (symbol)
38. Toward
40. Not off
41. Not of one's own accord
42. Look
43. Respiratory therapy (abbrev.)
45. Absence of breathing, usually temporary
46. Within normal limits (abbrev.)
47. Blow air from the lungs
48. Exist
49. Difficult breathing
51. Breathe air into the lungs
53. Not fast
54. Windpipe
56. Measure or distance of inspiration
57. Not she
58. Intermittent positive pressure breathing (abbrev.)
62. Inspire and expire
64. Medication
65. Inspire
67. Drug type that produces coughing

Down

6. Morphine sulfate (abbrev.)
7. Cough supressant
8. A pulmonary _____ carries oxygenated blood to the heart
9. Labored breathing that produces a snoring sound
12. Procedure to restore breathing
14. Implement placed over the nose and mouth to give oxygen
17. Name of bag-type equipment used for resuscitation
18. Blueness of tissues showing lack of oxygen
20. Frozen water
23. Actinon (symbol)
27. Between nasopharynx and laryngopharynx
30. Arouse
31. Percent of oxygen (abbrev.)
32. Machine used to maintain or control breathing
33. Pertaining to or involving the lungs
34. Humidification of oxygen provides this
38. Change position of the patient
39. Not deep
40. Gas needed to sustain life
44. Bronchodilator used in IPPB treatments
47. Every one
48. Brand name of respirator used for IPPB
50. Minute opening through which the skin breathes
52. Expire
54. Section of the body containing the heart, lungs, diaphragm, trachea, etc.
55. Composed of approximately 78% nitrogen, 21% oxygen, carbon dioxide, aqueous vapor, and traces of ammonia, helium, xenon, and other rare gases
59. Transfer of oxygen occurs in the capillary _____
60. Oral cavity; moisturizes inspired air
61. Upper respiratory infection (abbrev.)
63. Tender loving care (abbrev.)
66. Atropine sulfate (abbrev.)

TERMINOLOGY SEARCH 4: OPERATING ROOM SCHEDULE

This terminology search is an operating room schedule, with the names of patients and physicians deleted.

MCV OPERATING ROOM SCHEDULE   TUESDAY 12/ 6/83   TIME 11:03 14-MAR-84

RM	SER	START	A	LOC	DUR	PATIENT NAME	AGE	CHART #	X	OPERATION/COMMENT	SURGEONS	/	ANESTHESIA	ORDER
	X-RAY		G	M7	1:00	Patient A	17M	6056211		CT SCAN WO CONTRAST	Dr. A	/	Dr. B	A 1
2	VASC	07:40	G	M4GM	4:00	Patient B	63Y	7001611		EXP LAP; SMALL BOWEL OBSTRUCTIO	Dr. C	/	Dr. D	F A 1
2	VASC	11:11	G	M11E	4:00	Patient C	73Y	6083490	Y	RT FEMORAL-DISTAL BYPASS	Dr. E	/	Dr. F	F A 2
2	VASC	19:16	G	M4CI	2:00	Patient D	67Y	5648221		GREENFIELD FILTER	Dr. G	/	Dr. H	F U 3
3	PLAS	07:33	G	M9E	2:00	Patient E	70Y	5489488		EXC TUMOR, RT EAR WITH F.S.; PROB SKIN GRAFT; POSS 2ND STAGE EAR RECONSTRUCTION	Dr. I	/	Dr. J	F A 1
3	PLAS	10:15	G	M9E	2:00	Patient F	75Y	9320239		RESECTION & SKIN GRAFT, SQ CELL CA, DORSUM, RT HAND	Dr. K	/	Dr. L	F A 2
3	PLAS	12:16	G	M11W	4:00	Patient G	20Y	8042250	Y	REPAIR MANDIBULAR FRACTURE & MULTIPLE FACIAL FRACTURES	Dr. M	/	Dr. N	F A 3
4	VASC	07:32	G	W4E	3:00	Patient H	36Y	5318412		DRAINAGE LYMPHOCELE	Dr. O	/	Dr. P	F B 1
4	VASC	09:43	G	W15	2:00	Patient I	37Y	5449275		INSERTION TENCKHOFF CATH	Dr. Q	/	Dr. R	F B 2
5	GYN	07:32	G	M9C	5:00	Patient J	37Y	5634591		ANTERIOR EXENTERATION	Dr. S	/	Dr. T	F A 1
5	GYN	10:48	G	M9W	3:00	Patient K	69Y	6083090		EXPLORATORY LAPAROTOMY	Dr. U	/	Dr. V	F A 2
5	VASC	14:35	R	W4N	2:30	Patient L	73Y	5109359		REPAIR GORE-TEX, LT ARM	Dr. W	/	Dr. X	F T 3
6	PEDS	07:26	G	M7E	5:00	Patient M	11M	5646967	Y	ABDOMINAL-PERINEAL PULL-THRU	Dr. Y	/	Dr. Z	F A 1
7	ENT	07:31	G	M9E	1:30	Patient N	24Y	5496339		TONSILLECTOMY	Dr. a	/	Dr. b	F A 1
7	ENT	08:59	G	M9E	1:30	Patient O	23Y	5620994		TONSILLECTOMY	Dr. c	/	Dr. d	F A 2
7	ENT	10:45	G	M7CE	1:30	Patient P	16Y	5219730		TONSILLECTOMY	Dr. e	/	Dr. f	F A 3
7	ENT	12:25	G	W3S	1:30	Patient Q	24Y	4015972	Y	DIRECT LARYNGOSCOPY	Dr. g	/	Dr. h	F A 4
11	ENT	07:23	G	M9W	1:30	Patient R	55Y	5579558	Y	PANENDOSCOPY	Dr. i	/	Dr. j	F B 1
11	PEDS	09:58	G	M7E	1:45	Patient S	6M	6083780	Y	UPPER ENDOSCOPY	Dr. k	/	Dr. l	F B 2
11	ENT	12:00	G	M7CE	3:00	Patient T	17Y	5202121	Y	LT EXPLORATION TYMPANOTOMY	Dr. m	/	Dr. n	F B 3
12	ORAL	07:32	G	M7CE	2:30	Patient U	17Y	5628563		EXC RANULA, LT FOM	Dr. o	/	Dr. p	F A 1
12	ORAL	11:25	G	M9E	5:00	Patient V	70Y	5648331		MANDIBULAR OSTEOTOMY WITH ALLOPLASTIC AUGMENTATION	Dr. q	/	Dr. r	F A 2
15	CARD	07:37	L	W4S	2:00	Patient W	51Y	6074228		CARDIAC BIOPSY (FLUORO) X-RAY TECH NEEDED	Dr. s	/	Dr. t	F B 1
15	CARD	08:26	L	M4	2:00	Patient X	55Y	6082168		INSERTION TRANSVENOUS PACEMAKE	Dr. u	/	Dr. v	F B 2
17	ORTH	07:53	G	M4GS	4:00	Patient Y	81Y	5004930	Y	C1-C2 FUSION	Dr. w	/	Dr. x	F B 1
17	ORTH	13:42	G	W9E	3:00	Patient Z	29Y	6021374	Y	LT KNEE ARTHROSCOPY (TOURN)	Dr. y	/	Dr. z	F A 2
18	NEUR	08:00	G	M11W	5:00	Patient a	57Y	6083925		LT ECIC (MICROSCOPE)	Dr. AA	/	Dr. BB	F A 1
19	ORTH	07:46	G	W9S	3:00	Patient b	42Y	5141861	Y	LT TOTAL KNEE REPLACEMENT (FLUORO & TOURN) X-RAY TECH NEEDED	Dr. CC	/	DR. DD	F A 1
19	GEN	21:31	G	W3W	2:00	Patient c	19Y	5090131		APPENDECTOMY	Dr. EE	/	Dr. FF	F T 2
20	NEUR	07:17	G	M11W	4:00	Patient d	62Y	5598975	Y	LT POSTERIOR FOSSA EXPLORATION	Dr. GG	/	Dr. HH	F B 1
20	NEUR	14:27	G	M4	4:00	Patient e	71Y	8042262	Y	CRANIOTOMY FOR ANEURYSM	Dr. II	/	Dr. JJ	F B 2
21	ORTH	13:20	G	W9N	2:00	Patient f	91Y	6064862	Y	AUSTIN-MOORE PROSTHESIS, RT HIP	Dr. KK	/	Dr. LL	F A 1
22	UROL	07:45	G	M7SC	2:00	Patient g	17M	6055193		CYSTO; ENDOSCOPIC REMOVAL RENAL CALCULUS	Dr. MM	/	Dr. NN	F C 1
22	UROL	10:35	U		1:30	Patient h	55Y	7006446		NEPHROSTOGRAM	Dr. OO	/	Dr. PP	F T 2
23	UROL	08:25	U	M9C	1:30	Patient i	62Y	5632319		CYSTO, WASHINGS, POSS BLADDER BI	Dr. QQ	/	Dr. RR	F T 1
23	UROL	09:20	U	W15	1:30	Patient j	71Y	5533217		CYSTO;WASHINGS	Dr. SS	/	Dr. TT	F B 2
23	UROL	10:02	U	OP	1:30	Patient k	00D	5576942		CYSTO	Dr. UU	/	Dr. VV	F T 3
24	UROL	07:30	G	M10W	2:00	Patient l	27Y	5629960	Y	LT INGUINAL HERNIA REPAIR	Dr. WW	/	Dr. XX	F A 1
24	PEDS	10:55	G	M7E	1:30	Patient m	21M	5633695	Y	ESOPHAGEAL DILATATION	Dr. YY	/	Dr. ZZ	F A 2
25	OPHT	07:44	G	M9E	2:00	Patient n	24Y	6080492		ECCE,OD	Dr. aa	/	Dr. bb	F A 1
25	OPHT	09:46	L	M9E	3:00	Patient o	55Y	5076532		ECCE WITH POST CHAMBER IOL,OD	Dr. cc	/	Dr. dd	F A 2
25	OPHT	11:30	L	M9E	2:00	Patient p	49Y	6049154		ECCE WITH IOL,OD	Dr. ee	/	Dr. ff	F T 3
25	OPHT	13:25	L	M9E	2:30	Patient q	49Y	7005900		ECCE WITH POST CHAMBER IOL,OS	Dr. gg	/	Dr. hh	F A 4

COMMENTS CREATED——▶ 14-MAR-84   11:02:38

```
        CALL:
        CALL:
          OB:
          RR:
      POSTOP:
       OUTPT:
 COORDINATOR:
HOLDING AREA:
      TRAUMA:
    ACADEMIC:
     COMMENT:
```

Furnished by Medical College of Virginia Hospitals, Virginia Commonwealth University, Richmond, Virginia.

Substances

didn't do 1's

Substance: from Latin, meaning to exist

Word Element	Meaning	Aids to Learning	
		Illustrative Words	**Literal Meaning**
aero-, pneuma- pneumato- (Ā-e-rō) (NŪ-ma) (NŪ-ma-to)	air	aerodynamics, pneumatic	
amylo- (AM-i-lō)	starch	amylase	
enzymo- (EN-zī-mō)	enzyme		in yeast
fecalo- (FĒ-ka-lō)	feces		dregs
galacto-, lacto- (ga-LAK-tō) (LAK-tō)	milk	galaxy, lactic acid	
gluco-, glyco- saccharo- (GLOO-kō) (GLĪ-kō) (SAK-a-rō)	sugar	glycolysis, saccharin	gluco = sweet glyco = sweetness
-glia, colla- (GLĒ-a) (KOL-a)	glue	collagen	
halo-, sali- (HAL-ō) (SA-li)	salt	halogen, saline	
hidro-, sudori- (HID-rō) (SŪ-do-ri)	sweat		

| | Aids to Learning | | |
Word Element	Meaning	Illustrative Words	Literal Meaning
hormono- (HOR-mō-nō)	hormone		excite
hyalo, vitreo- (HĪ-a-lō) (VIT-rē-ō)	glass		
hydro-, aqueo- (HĪ-drō) (Ā-kwe-ō)	water	hydrotherapy, aqueous	
kal-	potassium		
kerato- (KER-a-tō)	keratin		horny
lipo-, adipo- (LIP-ō) (AD-i-pō)	fat	adipose tissue	
myxo-, muco- (MIK-sō) (MŪ-kō)	mucus		
natr-	sodium		
pharmaco- (FAR-ma-kō)	drug	pharmacy	
-plasm (plazm)	substance	cytoplasm	something formed
pyo-, puro- (PĪ-ō) (PŪ-rō)	pus	purulent, pyorrhea	
sebo-, -cer- (SEB-ō) (ser)	oil, wax	sebaceous	
semino- (SE-mi-nō)	semen	disseminate, seminary	seed
sialo-, ptyalo- (SĪ-a-lō) (TĪ-a-lō)	saliva		ptyalo = spittle
thio- (THĪ-ō)	sulfur		

WORDS USING THESE ELEMENTS

Record words given in class or encountered in your reading.

Word	Meaning

TEST YOUR KNOWLEDGE

Section A

Select from the list the substance to which each word element refers and write it in the blank.

1. Sebo- _oil_   saliva
2. Sialo- _saliva_   drug
3. Amylo- _starch_   sodium
4. Semino- _semen_   glass
5. Pharmaco- _drug_   starch
6. -plasm _substance_   keratin
7. Vitreo- _glass_   oil
8. Natr- _sodium_   substance
9. Kerato- _keratin_   semen
10. Kal- _potassium_   potassium

Section B

Give the definition of the following. Then give another word root with the same meaning.

1. Adipo- _Fat_   _lipo-_
2. Lacto- _milk_   _galacto-_
3. Halo-
4. Sudor-
5. Myxo-
6. Pyo-
7. Gluco- _sugar_   _sucro-_   _glyco-_
8. Aqueo- _water_   _hydro-_
9. -glia
10. Pneuma- _air_

Section C

Divide and define the following terms.

1. Hyaloid _resembling glass_
2. Pneumothorax _air chest_
3. Lactose _full of milk_
4. Seminiferous
5. Pyogenic _forming_
6. Pharmacology _study of drugs_
7. Hyperhidrosis _condition of_
8. Glycolysis _decomposition of sugar_
9. Neuroglia
10. Cytoplasm _cell_
11. Hypokalemia _less than normal potassium in the blood_
12. Galactosemia _sugar in the blood_
13. Collagenous _resembling glue_
14. Sialolith _stone of salt_
15. Lipolytic _destruction of fat_

Section D

Complete the following terms.

1. _____ sali gen   (chemical element) producing a salt

2. _____ pyo rrhea   flow of pus

3. Poly _____   many sugars

4. _____ cyte   cell (that makes) keratin

5. _____ lysin   enzyme that destroys wax

6. _____ urea   urea in which (oxygen is replaced by) sulfur

7. _____ ferous   bearing sweat

8. Poly _____   much saliva

9. Hyper _____ emia   more than normal sodium in blood

10. _____ genesis   formation of sugar

11. _____ poiesis   formation of hormones

12. _____ uria   enzymes in the urine

13. _____ Fecal lith   stone in the feces

14. _____ edema   mucous swelling

15. _____ osis   fat condition (obesity)

16. _____ lipo rrheic   pertaining to a flow of oil

17. _____ colitis   inflammation of colon with mucus

18. _____ sal ine   salty

19. _____ neogenesis   formation of new sugar

20. _____ pneumo cardia   air in the heart

Answers to Lesson 18—page 233

141

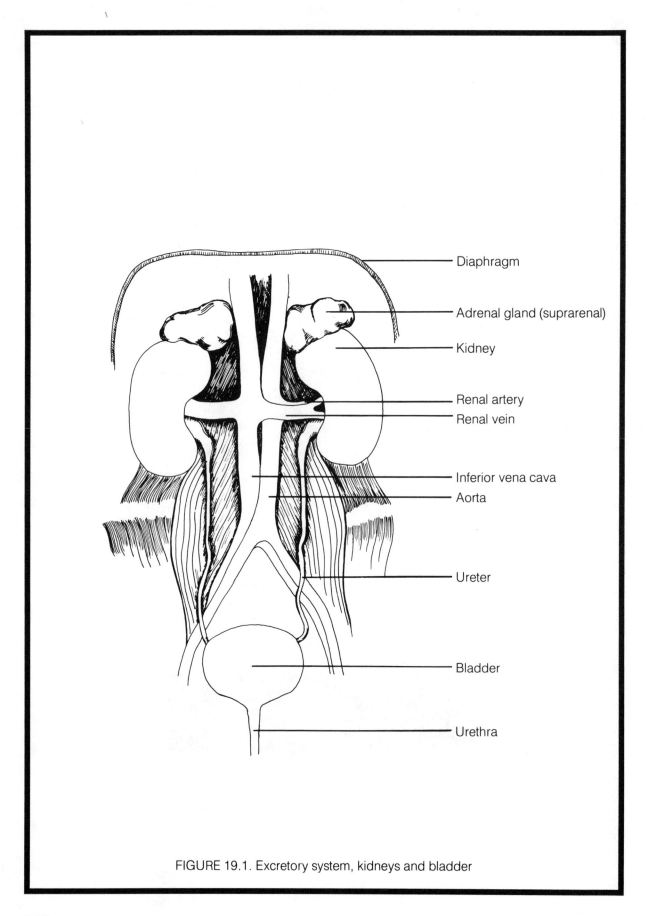

FIGURE 19.1. Excretory system, kidneys and bladder

Diaphragm

Adrenal gland (suprarenal)

Kidney

Renal artery

Renal vein

Inferior vena cava

Aorta

Ureter

Bladder

Urethra

LESSON 19

Urogenital Systems

Uro: from Greek, meaning urine
Genital: from Latin, meaning belonging to birth

The vital function of the urinary system is to insure that the chemical composition of the blood and other body fluids is kept within a narrow range. The accumulation of excess chemicals, the production of dissolved waste, and the presence of toxic substances all require an organ that will selectively remove from the blood those substances that should be excreted from the body and retain those that are needed. The *kidney*, which does this, has an enormous number of tubules called *nephrons* that are intimately associated with blood capillaries. The product of several complex exchanges between these two is urine. Urine drips from the tubules into the *renal pelvis*, and is moved by peristalsis through the *ureter* to the *bladder*. The *urethra* is the passage for its release to the outside of the body.

By means of the female and male reproductive systems, a new organism develops from the fusion of two *gametes*: an egg and a sperm. These reproductive cells are produced in ovary and testis, which are called *gonads*. Sperm from the *testis*, which is situated in a skin pouch called the *scrotum*, accumulate in the *epididymis* until emission. They are then moved by muscular action through the *vas deferens*, *ejaculatory duct*, and *urethra* to the external opening at the tip of the penis. The *prostate* and other glands secrete the fluid *semen*, in which the sperm leave the body.

The egg or *ovum* leaving the *ovary* enters the *uterine* or *fallopian tube*, where it may be fertilized if sperm are present. During the succeeding days, the developing embryo is moved to the *uterus*, where it implants in the *endometrium*. The *placenta*, a combination of maternal and fetal tissue, is constructed so that the blood of each is exposed to the other over a large surface, permitting acquisition by the fetus of all necessary substances and the release of fetal waste to maternal blood. The fetus completes its development within the fluid-filled *amnion*; birth occurs through the *vagina*.

Combining form	Anatomical Usage	Aids to Learning	
		Common Name	Literal Meaning
Urinary System			
nephro-, reno- (NEF-rō) (RĒ-nō)	kidney		
pyelo- (PĪ-e-lō)	kidney pelvis		pelvis = basin
uretero- (ū-RE-ter-ō)	ureter		
cysto-, vesico- (SIS-tō) (VES-i-kō)	bladder		cyst = sac
urethro- (ū-RE-thrō)	urethra		

143

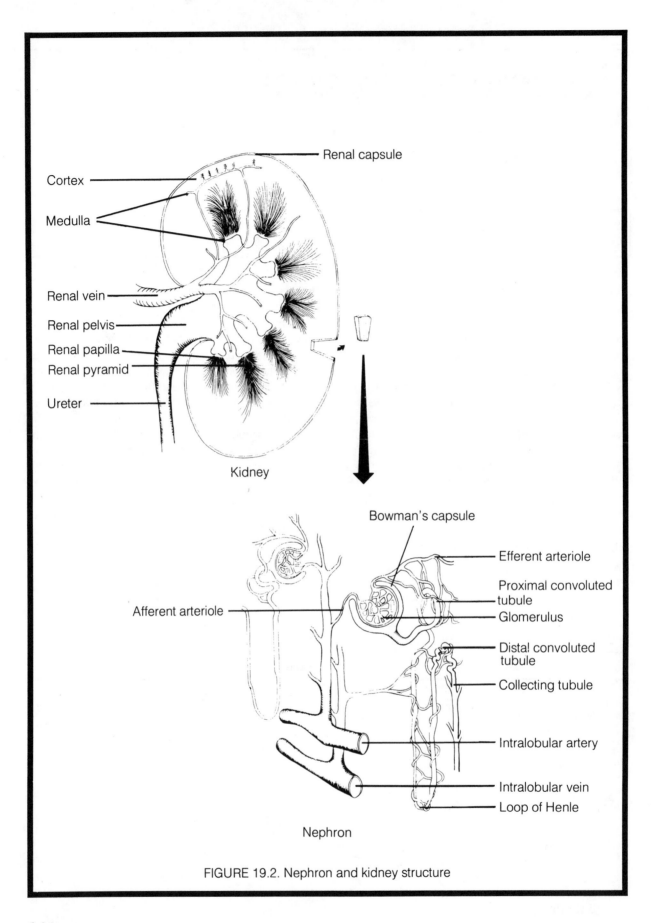

Renal capsule

Cortex

Medulla

Renal vein

Renal pelvis

Renal papilla

Renal pyramid

Ureter

Kidney

Bowman's capsule

Efferent arteriole

Proximal convoluted tubule

Afferent arteriole

Glomerulus

Distal convoluted tubule

Collecting tubule

Intralobular artery

Intralobular vein

Loop of Henle

Nephron

FIGURE 19.2. Nephron and kidney structure

144

	Aids to Learning		
Combining Form	**Anatomical Usage**	**Common Name**	**Literal Meaning**
Reproductive System (Reproduce: from Latin, meaning lead forth again)			
♀	female		mirror of Venus
gyneco- (JIN-e-kō)	woman		woman = out of man
oophoro-, ovario- (ō-OF-ō-rō) (ō-VĀ-rē-ō)	ovary		oophoro = eggbearer
oo-, ovo- (Ō-Ō) (Ō-vō)	ovum	egg	
salpingo- (sal-PING-gō)	uterine tube	fallopian tube	trumpet
hystero-, metro- **utero-** (HIS-ter-ō) (Ū-ter-ō)	uterus	womb	
colpo-, vagino- (KOL-pō) (VAJ-i-nō)	vagina	birth canal	sheath
thelo-, mamilli- (THĒ-lō) (ma-MIL-i)	nipple		
masto-, mammo- (MAS-tō) (MAM-ō)	breast		
vulva, episio- (e-PIZ-ē-ō)	area of external openings	external genitalia	
placento- (pla-SEN-tō)	placenta	afterbirth	flat cake
amnio- (AM-nē-ō)	amnion	bag of waters	bowl
♂	male		arrow of Mars
andro- (AN-drō)	man		
orchido-, orchio- **testi** (OR-ki-dō) (OR-kē-ō)	testis		testis = witness

145

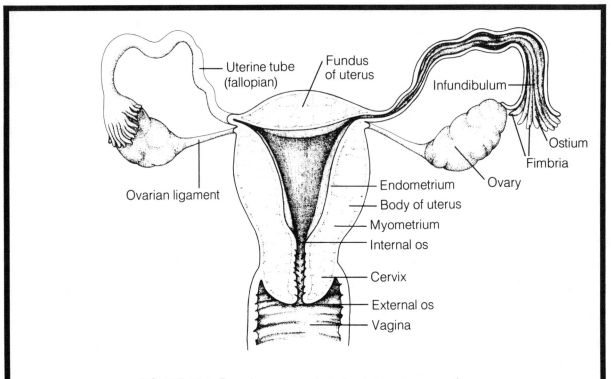

FIGURE 19.3. Female ovary and uterine tube, uterus section

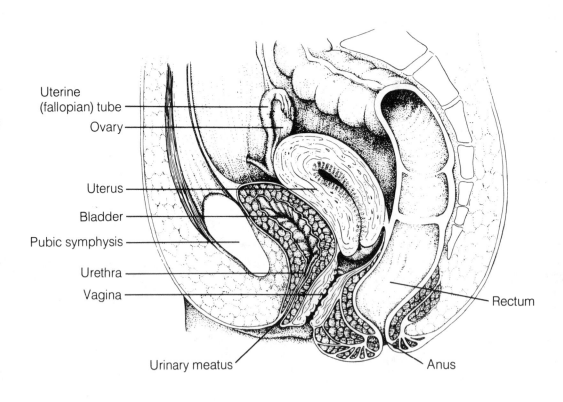

FIGURE 19.4. Female reproductive system, sagittal section

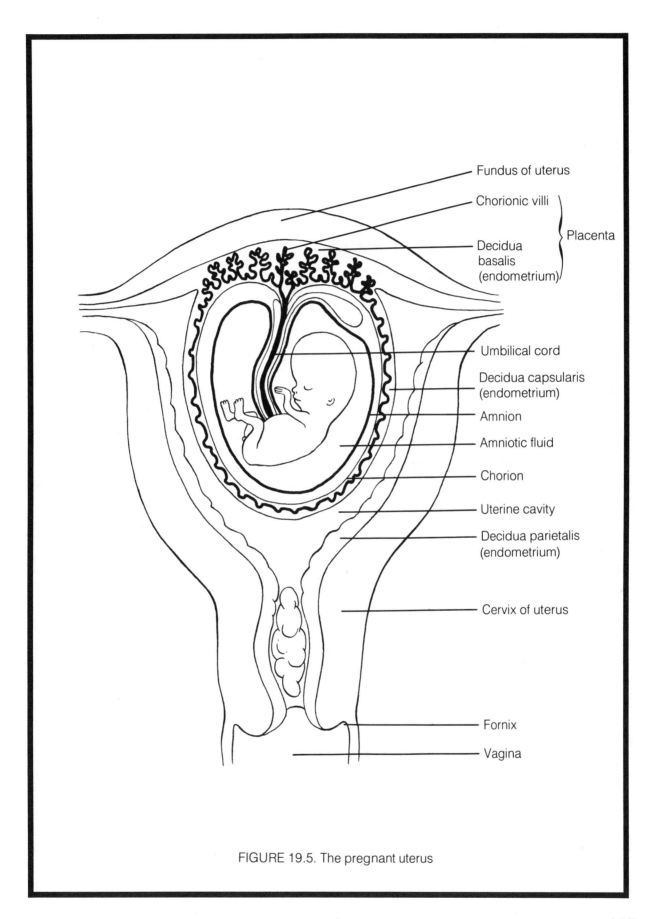

Fundus of uterus

Chorionic villi

Placenta

Decidua basalis (endometrium)

Umbilical cord

Decidua capsularis (endometrium)

Amnion

Amniotic fluid

Chorion

Uterine cavity

Decidua parietalis (endometrium)

Cervix of uterus

Fornix

Vagina

FIGURE 19.5. The pregnant uterus

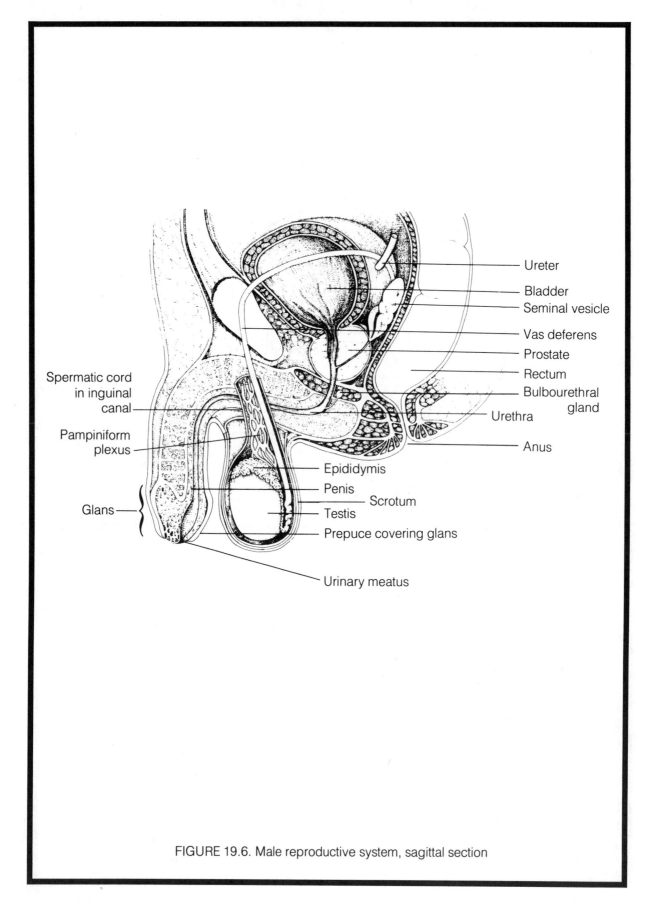

Ureter

Bladder

Seminal vesicle

Vas deferens

Prostate

Rectum

Bulbourethral gland

Urethra

Anus

Spermatic cord in inguinal canal

Pampiniform plexus

Glans

Epididymis

Penis

Scrotum

Testis

Prepuce covering glans

Urinary meatus

FIGURE 19.6. Male reproductive system, sagittal section

	Aids to Learning		
Combining Form	Anatomical Usage	Common Name	Literal Meaning

<table>
<tr><td colspan="4" align="center">Reproductive System (Reproduce: from Latin, meaning lead forth again)</td></tr>
<tr><td>scroto-
(SKRŌ-tō)</td><td>scrotum</td><td></td><td>bag</td></tr>
<tr><td>spermato-
(SPER-ma-tō)</td><td>sperm</td><td></td><td>seed</td></tr>
<tr><td>semino-
(SE-min-ō)</td><td>semen</td><td>ejaculate (substance)</td><td>seed</td></tr>
<tr><td>phallo-
(FAL-ō)</td><td>penis</td><td></td><td></td></tr>
<tr><td>vaso-
(VAS-ō)</td><td>vas deferens</td><td>sperm duct</td><td>deferens = carry away</td></tr>
<tr><td>epididymo-
(ep-i-DID-i-mō)</td><td>epididymis</td><td></td><td>upon twins</td></tr>
<tr><td>prostato-
(pros-TAT-ō)</td><td>prostate gland</td><td></td><td>stand before</td></tr>
<tr><td>preputio-
(pre-PŪ-shē-ō)</td><td>prepuce</td><td>foreskin</td><td></td></tr>
<tr><td colspan="4" align="center">Both Sexes</td></tr>
<tr><td>gono-
(GON-ō)</td><td>gonad</td><td>reproductive organ</td><td>seed</td></tr>
<tr><td>gamo-
(GAM-ō)</td><td>gamete</td><td>reproductive cell</td><td>wife, husband</td></tr>
<tr><td>perineo-
(per-i-NĒ-ō)</td><td>perineum</td><td>area of external openings</td><td></td></tr>
</table>

WORDS USING THESE ELEMENTS

Record words given in class or encountered in your reading.

Word	Meaning
_____	_____
_____	_____
_____	_____
_____	_____
_____	_____
_____	_____
_____	_____
_____	_____
_____	_____
_____	_____
_____	_____

TEST YOUR KNOWLEDGE

Section A

Divide and define the following terms.

1. Pyelonephritis _inflammation_
2. Urocystoclysis _irrigation_
3. Urethrostenosis _infection in urethra_
4. Amniocentesis _puncture amnion_
5. Myometrium _uterus muscle_
6. Oogenesis _formation of ovum (egg)_
7. Orchidopexy _fixation of the testis_
8. Phallic _pertaining to penis_
9. Perineorrhaphy _suture in perineum_
10. Transurethral _pertaining to around the urethra_
11. Spermatolysis _destruction of sperm_
12. Scrotocele _herniation of the scrotum_
13. Mamillary _pertaining to breast_
14. Epithelium (which has come to refer to all surface tissue) _____

150

15. Mastocarcinoma _cancer tumor in the breast_
16. Salpingocyesis _pregnancy in the uterine tube_
17. Gynecomastia (occurs in males) _condition (Abnormal) of women breast_
18. Ureterolith _stone in ureter_
19. Suprarenal _pertaining to above the kidney_
20. Hysterosalpingo-oophorectomy _removal of ovary, uterine tube, & uterus_

Section B

Construct terms for the following definitions.

1. Flow from the reproductive organs _gono rrhea_
2. Resembling a breast _mammiloid_
3. Inflammaton of the epididymis _Epididymo itis_
4. Removal of (part of) the vas deferens _vas Ectomy_
5. Process of recording the bladder _cysto graphy_
6. Inflammation of the uterine tubes and ovaries _salpingo-oophoritis_
7. Specialist in the study of women _gynecologist_
8. Incision into the ureter _ureter tomy_
9. Pain in the bladder _cysto algia_
10. Dilatation of the vagina _colpo Ectasis_

Section C

Complete the following definitions.

1. Poly/andr/y   many _men_
2. Vesic/o/perine/al   pertaining to _bladder_ and _perineum_
3. Preputi/o/tomy   incision into the _prepuce_
4. Gynec/o/genic   producing _woman_ (characteristics)
5. Phall/oncus   tumor of the _penis_
6. Prostat/o/megaly   enlargement of the _prostate gland_
7. Salping/o/graphy   recording of the _uterine tubes_
8. Endometri/osis   abnormal condition of tissue usually _inside the uterus_
9. Amnio/rrhexis   rupture of the _amnion_
0. Epi/nephr/os   (gland located) _upon the kidney_

Section D

Complete the following terms.

1. _____ _gon_ ad   reproductive organ

2. Poly _thelo_ _____   many nipples

3. _____plasty   repair of the vulva

4. _____ itis   inflammation of vulva and vagina

5. _____ cele   herniation of the perineum

6. _____ atresia   imperforation of the urethra

7. A _____   without breasts

8. _____ _oo_ kinesia   movement of the egg

9. _____ oma   tumor of placenta

10. _____plication   folding of renal pelvis

Answers to Lesson 19—page 234

Following are diagrams of the urinary and reproductive systems. On each label line, write in the name of the part.

Write each combining form on the appropriate label line.

Adreno-, suprareno-
Cysto-
Nephro-, reno-
Phreno-
Uretero-
Urethro-

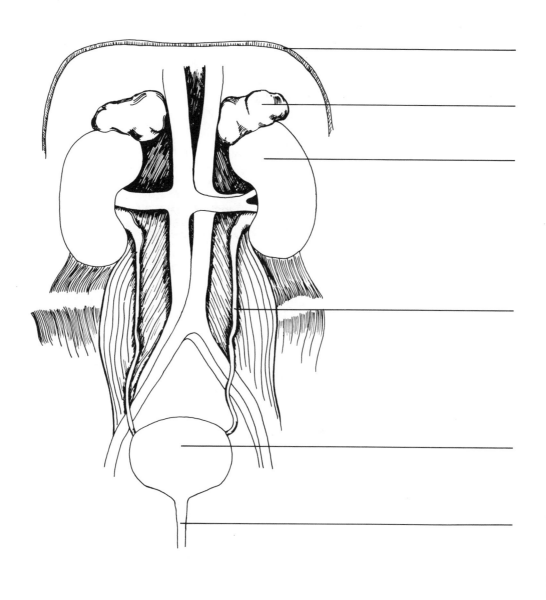

FIGURE 19.7. Excretory system, kidneys and bladder

Write each term or combining form on the appropriate label line.

Afferent arteriole   Intra- (use twice)
Cortex   Medulla
Distal   Papilla
Efferent arteriole   Proximal
                      Pyelo-
                      Uretero-

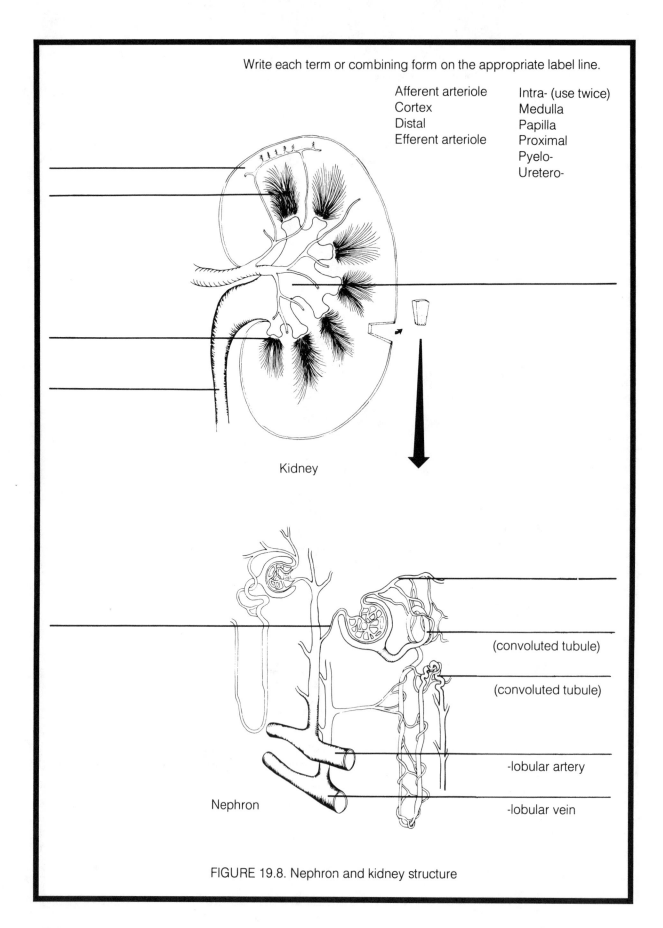

Kidney

Nephron

(convoluted tubule)

(convoluted tubule)

-lobular artery

-lobular vein

FIGURE 19.8. Nephron and kidney structure

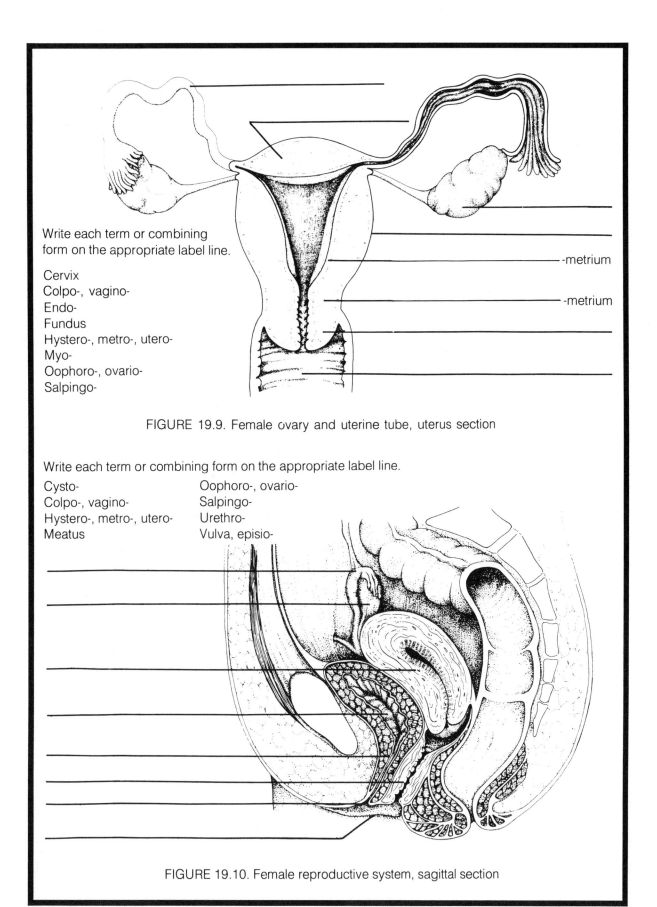

Write each term or combining
form on the appropriate label line.

Cervix
Colpo-, vagino-
Endo-
Fundus
Hystero-, metro-, utero-
Myo-
Oophoro-, ovario-
Salpingo-

-metrium

-metrium

FIGURE 19.9. Female ovary and uterine tube, uterus section

Write each term or combining form on the appropriate label line.

Cysto-   Oophoro-, ovario-
Colpo-, vagino-   Salpingo-
Hystero-, metro-, utero-   Urethro-
Meatus   Vulva, episio-

FIGURE 19.10. Female reproductive system, sagittal section

Write each term or combining form on the appropriate label line.

Amnio-
Cervix
Chorion
Colpo-, vagino-
Endometrium
Fundus
Parietalis
Placento-
Salpingo-
Umbilical

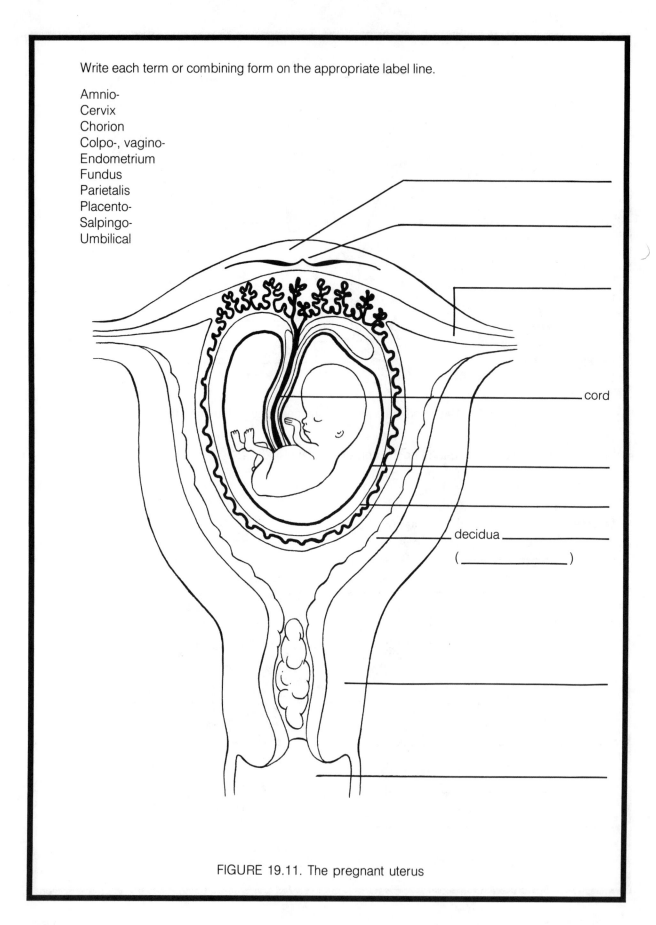

cord

decidua

(_____)

FIGURE 19.11. The pregnant uterus

Write each term or combining form on the appropriate label line.

Ano-
Bulbourethral
Cysto-
Epididymo-
Inguinal
Meatus

Orchido-, testi-
Phallo-
Preputio-
Prostato-
Recto-
Scroto-

Seminal vesicle
Spermatic
Uretero-
Urethro-
Vaso-

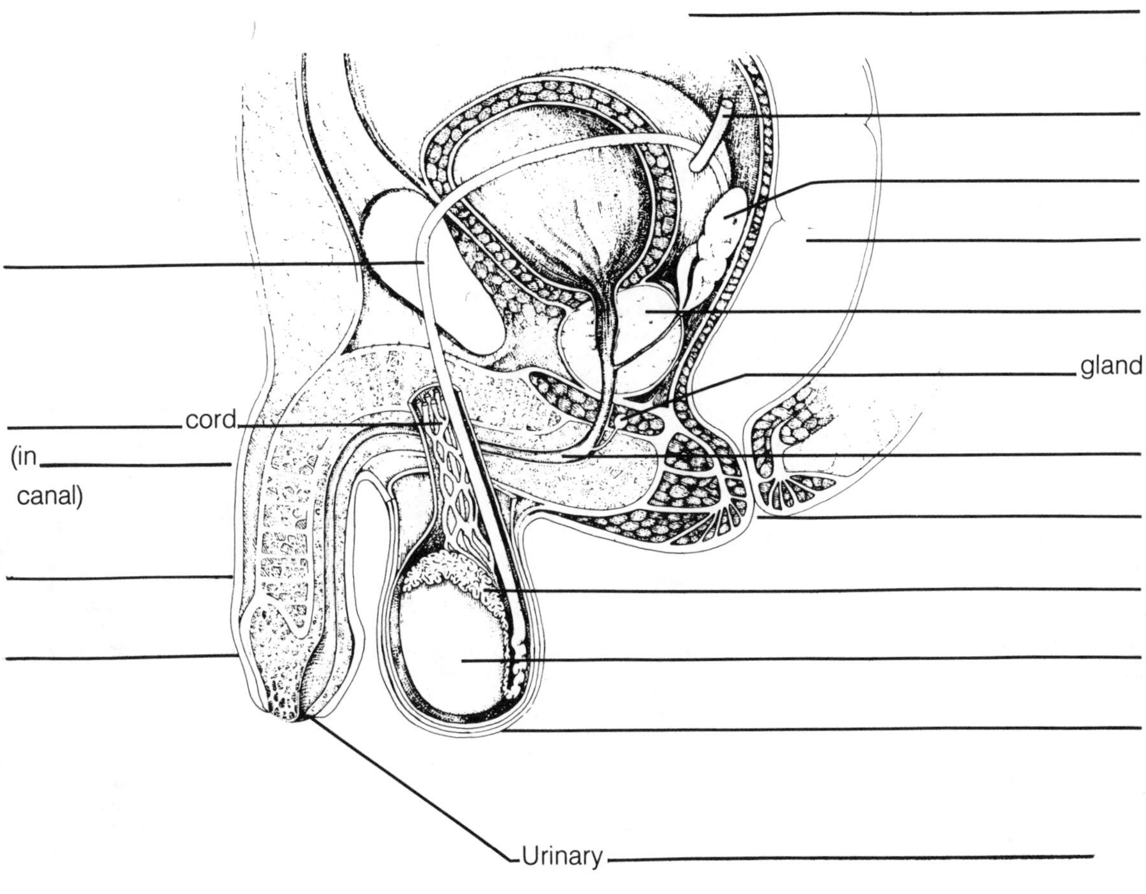

_____ cord

(in _____
canal)

_____ gland

_____ Urinary _____

FIGURE 19.12. Male reproductive system, sagittal section

157

The *Nurses Research Library* consists of a number of volumes containing information necessary for the professional nurse. This excerpt is from the volume *Diseases*.

The signs and symptoms of renal vein thrombosis vary with the speed of onset. Do you know what to look for?

RENAL VEIN THROMBOSIS

JUNE L. STARK, RN
Critical Care Instructor
Tufts-New England Medical Center
Boston, Massachusetts

RENAL VEIN THROMBOSIS, clotting in the renal vein, results in renal congestion, engorgement, and possibly infarction. Such thrombosis may affect both kidneys and may occur in a chronic or an acute form. Chronic thrombosis usually impairs renal function, causing nephrotic syndrome. Acute thrombosis that causes extensive damage may precipitate rapidly fatal renal infarction. If thrombosis affects both kidneys, prognosis is poor. However, less severe thrombosis that affects only one kidney, or gradual progression that allows development of collateral circulation may preserve partial renal function.

Causes

Renal vein thrombosis often results from a tumor that obstructs the renal vein (usually hypernephroma). Other causes include thrombophlebitis of the inferior vena cava or blood vessels of the legs, congestive heart failure, and periarteritis. In infants, renal vein thrombosis usually follows diarrhea that causes severe dehydration. Chronic renal vein thrombosis is often a complication of other glomerulopathic diseases, such as amyloidosis, diabetic nephropathy, and membranoproliferative glomerulonephritis.

Signs and symptoms

Clinical features of renal vein thrombosis vary with speed of onset. Rapid onset of venous obstruction produces severe lumbar pain and tenderness in the epigastric region and the costovertebral angle. Other characteristic features include fever, leukocytosis, pallor, hematuria, proteinuria, peripheral edema, and when the obstruction is bilateral, oliguria and other uremic

signs. The kidneys enlarge and become easily palpable. Hypertension is unusual, but may develop.

Gradual onset causes symptoms of nephrotic syndrome. Peripheral edema is possible, but pain is generally absent. Other clinical signs include proteinuria, hypoalbuminemia, and hyperlipemia.

Infants with this disease have enlarged kidneys, oliguria, and renal insufficiency that may progress to acute or chronic renal failure.

Diagnosis

• *Intravenous pyelography* provides reliable diagnostic evidence. In acute renal vein thrombosis, the kidneys appear enlarged and excretory function diminishes. Contrast medium gives necrotic renal tissue a smudged appearance. In chronic thrombosis, the X-ray may show ureteral indentations that result from collateral venous channels. Renal arteriography and biopsy may also confirm the diagnosis.
• *Urinalysis* reveals gross or microscopic hematuria, proteinuria (more than 2 grams/day in chronic disease), casts, and oliguria.
• *Blood studies* show leukocytosis, hypoalbuminemia, and hyperlipemia.

Treatment

Treatment is most effective for gradual thrombosis that affects only one kidney. Anticoagulant therapy (heparin or warfarin) may prove helpful, particularly if it's long term. To be effective, surgery must be performed within 24 hours of thrombosis, but even then it may have limited success since thrombi often extend into the small veins. Extensive intrarenal bleeding may necessitate nephrectomy.

Patients who survive acute thrombosis with extensive renal damage develop nephrotic syndrome and require treatment for renal failure, such as dialysis and possibly transplantation. Some infants with renal vein thrombosis recover completely following heparin therapy or surgical removal of the thrombus; others suffer irreversible kidney damage.

Nursing intervention

• Assess renal function and provide appropriate emotional support, particularly for parents of an affected infant.
• Monitor vital signs, intake and output, daily weight, and electrolytes. Administer diuretics for edema, as ordered, and enforce dietary restrictions, such as limited sodium and potassium intake.
• Monitor closely for signs of pulmonary emboli (chest pain, dyspnea).
• If heparin is given by continuous intravenous infusion, dilute the drug and administer it by infusion pump or controller, so the patient receives the least amount necessary. Monitor partial thromboplastin time frequently to determine the response.
• During anticoagulant therapy, watch for and report signs of bleeding, such as tachycardia, hypotension, hematuria, bleeding from nose or gums, ecchymoses, petechiae, and tarry stools. Instruct the patient on maintenance warfarin therapy to use an electric razor and a soft toothbrush, and to avoid trauma. Suggest that he wear a medical identification bracelet, and tell him to avoid aspirin, which aggravates bleeding tendencies. Stress the need for close medical follow-up.

From the NURSE'S REFERENCE LIBRARY volume *Diseases*.

Miscellaneous Word Elements 2

Miscellaneous: from Latin, meaning little mixture

Word Element	Meaning	Aids to Learning	
		Illustrative Words	Literal Meaning
acro- (AK-rō)	extremity	acrobat	high, tip
ankylo- (ANG-ki-lō)	stiffness, adhesion		
baro-	pressure	barometer	weight
-bol-	throw	metabolism, embolus	
chiasma (kī-AS-ma)	crossing point		from Greek letter chi
chorio- (KŌ-rē-ō)	membrane	chorion	
-cid- (sīd)	kill	homicide	
circum-	around	circumference	
cocco- (KOK-ō)	spherical cell	staphylococcus	berry
crypto-	hidden	cryptic	
-erg-	work	energy	
follicle (FOL-li-kl)	small sac or cavity		little bag
foramen (fo-RĀ-men)	opening		

		Aids to Learning	
Word Element	**Meaning**	**Illustrative Words**	**Literal Meaning**
fornix (FOR-niks)	arch		
fossa (FOS-a)	depressed area		trench
fovea (FŌ-vē-a)	pit		
geri- , geronto- (JER-ē) (jer-ON-tō)	old age	gerontology, geriatrics	
-gnosis (NŌ-sis)	knowledge	diagnosis, agnostic	
idio- (ID-ē-ō)	one's own	idiosyncrasy	peculiar
infundibulum (in-fun-DIB-ū-lum)	funnel-shaped tube		
insula (IN-sū-la)	isolated	insular	island
lamella (la-MEL-a)	thin layer		
lamina (LAM-i-na)	layer	laminate	
lumen (LOO-men)	cavity of hollow organ	illuminate	light
myco- (MĪ-kō)	fungus	streptomycin	
necro- , mort- (NEK-rō)	death	necrology, immortal	
nucleo- (NŪ-klē-ō)	central structure	nucleus	nut, kernel
pedo- (PĒ-dō)	child	pediatrics	
-phon- (fōn)	sound	symphony, telephone	voice
radiculo- (ra-DIK-ū-lō)	root	radical	

Word Element	Meaning	Illustrative Words	Literal Meaning
ruga (ROO-ga)	fold	corrugated	wrinkle
staphylo- (STAF-i-lō)	cluster	staphylococcus	bunch of grapes
stereo-	solid	stereophonic, cholesterol	
-sthenia (STHĒ-nē-a)	strength		
stratum (STRAT-um)	layer	stratified	
stria (STRĪ-a)	stripe	striated	
taxo-	order	syntax, taxidermy	arrangement
toxico- (TOK-si-kō)	poison	toxicology, toxemia	bow (and arrow)
tricho- , pilo- (TRIK-ō) (PĪ-lō)	hair	trichinosis, depilatory	
xero- (ZĒ-rō)	dry	Xerox	

WORDS USING THESE ELEMENTS

Record words given in class or encountered in your reading.

Word	Meaning
_____	_____
_____	_____
_____	_____
_____	_____
_____	_____
_____	_____
_____	_____

TEST YOUR KNOWLEDGE

Section A

Select from the list the meaning of the following anatomical terms and write them in the blank.

1. Fovea _____ *pit* _____ depressed area

2. Insula _____ *isolated part* _____ pit

3. Fornix _____ *Arch* _____ cavity of hollow organ

4. Chiasma _____ *crossing point* _____ small sac

5. Ruga _____ *internal fold* _____ opening

6. Fossa _____ *depressed area* _____ internal fold

7. Foramen _____ *opening* _____ thin layer

8. Lamella _____ *thin layer* _____ arch

9. Follicle _____ *small sac* _____ crossing point

10. Lumen _____ *cavity of hollow organ* _____ isolated part

Section B

Divide and define the following terms.

1. Toxemia _____ *condition of poison in blood* _____

2. Idiopathic _____ *pertaining to one's own disease* _____

3. Dermatomycosis _____

4. Geriatric _____ *pertaining to old age* _____

5. Ankylodactylia _____ *condition of stiff digits* _____

6. Bactericidal _____ *pertaining to killing bacteria* _____

7. Myasthenia _____ *weakness of muscle* _____

8. Xerophthalmia _____

9. Prognosis _____ *before knowledge* _____

10. Choroid _____ *resembling a membrane* _____

11. Radiculotomy _____

12. Cryptorchidism _____ *condition of hidden testes* _____

13. Circumcision _____

14. Stratified _____

15. Striated _____

16. Spermicidal _____ *pertaining to killing sperm* _____

17. Cholesterol _____

162

18. Necrotic _pertaing to dEath_

19. Hyperbaric _pertaing to more than normal pressure_

20. Meningococci _spherical cell in meninges_

Section C

Construct terms for the following definitions.

1. Fear of death _necrophobia_

2. Cluster of spherical cells _staphylococci_

3. Without hair _Apilo_

4. Instrument to measure pressure _baro meter_

5. Without order _Ataxic_

6. Lack of nerve strength _neuroAsthenia_

7. Record of work _Ergogram_

8. Across the cavity of a hollow organ _lumen_

9. Around the isolated part _peri insula_

10. Poison from fungi _mycotoxoid_

11. Enlargement of extremities _megaly_

12. Study of old age _gerontology_

13. Tumor of the infundibulum _infundibul..._

14. Opening between vertebrae _v foramen_

15. Pertaining to stopping (growth of) fungi _mycocidal   mycostatic_

16. Specialist in children's teeth _pedodentist_ notKill

Answers to Lesson 20—page 236

Qualities

Quality: from Latin, meaning of what kind

Combining Form	Meaning	Aids to Learning Illustrative Words
		Colors
leuko-, leuco- (LOO-kō)	white	leukemia
melano- (MEL-a-nō)	black	melancholy
xantho-, luteo- (ZAN-thō) (LOO-tē-ō)	yellow	
cirrho- (SIR-rō)	yellow-orange	cirrhosis
purpuri- (PUR-pū-ri)	purple	
cyano- (SĪ-a-nō)	blue	cyanotic, cyanide
polio-	gray	poliomyelitis
glauco- (GLAW-kō)	greenish-gray, silvery	glaucoma
erythro- (e-RITH-rō)	red	erythrocyte

		Aids to Learning
Combining Form	**Meaning**	**Illustrative Words**
Size, Shape, Texture		
micro-	small	microbe
macro-, megalo- (MAK-rō) (MEG-a-lō)	large	megalopolis, macromolecule
dolicho- (DOL-i-kō)	long	
brachy- (BRAK-ē)	short	
lepto-	thin	
pachy- (PAK-ē)	thick	pachyderm
steno-	narrow	stenographer
eury- (Ū-rē)	wide	
platy- (PLAT-ē)	flat, broad	platypus
ortho-, recto-	straight	orthodontist, direct
scolio-, strepto- (SKŌ-lē-ō)	twisted	scoliosis, streptococcus
trach-, trachy- (TRAK) (TRAK-ē)	rough	trachea
leio- (LĪ-ō)	smooth	
bary- (BAR-i)	heavy	baritone
oxy- (OK-sē)	sharp, acid, fast	oxygen

WORDS USING THESE ELEMENTS

Record words given in class or encountered in your reading.

Word	Meaning
_____	_____
_____	_____
_____	_____
_____	_____
_____	_____
_____	_____
_____	_____
_____	_____
_____	_____
_____	_____
_____	_____
_____	_____
_____	_____

TEST YOUR KNOWLEDGE

Section A

Select the color for each combining form and write it in the blank.

1. Cyano- _____blue_____ black
2. Polio- _____gray_____ purple
3. Melano- _____black_____ red
4. Xantho- _____yellow_____ blue
5. Leuco- _____white_____ yellow
6. Glauco- _____greenish-gray, silvery_____ gray
7. Cirrho- _____yellow-orange_____ yellow-orange
8. Luteo- _____white yellow_____ greenish-gray, silvery
9. Purpuri _____purple_____ white
10. Erythro- _____red_____

Section B

Select the size, shape, or texture referred to by each combining form and write it in the blank.

1. Pachy- _____thick_____   straight
2. Ortho- _____straight_____   smooth
3. Macro- _____large_____   rough
4. Eury- _____wide_____   thick
5. Leio- _____smooth_____   small
6. Trachy- _____rough_____   large
7. Brachy- _____short_____   short
8. Recto- _____straight_____   wide
9. Micro- _____small_____   twisted
10. Scolio- _____twisted_____

Section C

Divide and define the following terms.

1. Brachydactyly _____condition of short digit_____
2. Microphthalmia _____condition of_____
3. Melanoma _____tumor black_____
4. Corpus luteum _____
5. Macrophage _____large_____
6. Dolichocephalic _____pertaining to long head_____
7. Leukocytosis _____condition of white cells_____
8. Cyanosis _____condition of blue_____
9. Orthodontist _____specialist in straight teeth_____
10. Platyrrhine _____broad flat_____
11. Rectus abdominis _____
12. Poliomyelitis _____inflammation of gray muscle_____
13. Scoliorachitis _____inflammation_____
14. Euryopia _____wide vision_____
15. Leiodermia _____condition of smooth skin_____
16. Erythrocytopoiesis _____formation of red cells_____

Section D

Construct terms for the following.

1. Tumor of smooth muscle _leiomyoma_
2. Pertaining to white skin _leuko-dermatic_
3. Tumor of thin meninges _leptomeningoma_
4. Disease of the gray (matter) of the brain _polioencephalpathy_
5. Greenish-gray tumor (increased pressure of fluid in eye) _glaucoma_
6. Deficiency of red (cells in blood) _Erythropenia_
7. Large teeth _macro_
8. Black vomit _melano_
9. Blue vision _cyanoptia_
10. Short lips _brachylabia_
11. Having an affinity for acid (dye) _oxyphilic_
12. Pertaining to twisted spherical cells _streptococceal_
13. Rough tumor (eye disease) _trachoma_
14. Pertaining to "straight child" _orthopedic_
15. Thick nails _pachyonchyno_
16. Small breasts _micromammary_   _mast_
17. Pertaining to wide head _eurycephalic_
18. Yellow color
19. Flat feet _podoplaty_
20. Narrow mouth
21. Large hands _macro_   _-chiro_

Answers to Lesson 21—page 237

169

Quantities

Quantity: from Latin, meaning how great

		Aids to Learning
Combining Form	**Meaning**	**Illustrative Words**
mono-, uni-	one	monorail, universe
haplo-	single	
di-, bi-	two	dipole, bifocals
diplo-	double	diploma
tri-	three	trio
triplo-	triple	
tetra-, quadri-	four	quadruplets, tetrachloride
deca- (DEK-a)	ten	decade
deci- (DES-i)	one-tenth	decibel
hecto- (HEK-tō)	hundred	hectare
centi- (SEN-ti)	one-hundredth	century
kilo- (KIL-ō)	thousand	kilogram
milli- (MIL-ē)	one-thousandth	millipede

Combining Form	Meaning	Illustrative Words
poly-, multi-	many, much	polygamy, multiply
nulli-	none	nullify
oligo- (OL-i-gō)	few, little	
pan-, pant-	all	panacea, pantomime, Panamerican
hypo-, meio-, mio- (MĪ-ō)	less	hypothyroid, meiosis
hyper-, pleo- (PLĒ-ō)	more	hyperactive
hemi-, semi-	half	hemisphere, semicircular

WORDS USING THESE ELEMENTS

Record words given in class or encountered in your reading.

Word	Meaning
_____	_____
_____	_____
_____	_____
_____	_____
_____	_____
_____	_____
_____	_____
_____	_____
_____	_____
_____	_____
_____	_____

TEST YOUR KNOWLEDGE

Section A

Give the meaning of the following.

1. Diplo- _double_
2. Deci- _$\frac{1}{1000}$_
3. Centi- _$\frac{1}{100}$_
4. Poly- _many_
5. Pan- _All_
6. Mono- _one_
7. Pleo- _more_
8. Semi- _half_
9. Triplo- _triple_
10. Quadri- _Four_

Section B

Give the word root for the following words.

1. Thousand _Kilo_
2. Less _hypo   meio   mio_
3. Half _semi   hemi_
4. Single _haplo_
5. Three _tri_
6. None _nulli_
7. Few _oligo_
8. Two _di   bi_
9. Hundred _hecto_
10. All _pan   pant_

Section C

Divide and define the following terms.

1. Meiosis _____
2. Triploblastic _____
3. Hemiplegia _half paralyzied_
4. Nulliparous _pertaining to not giving birth_
5. Pancytopenia _formation of all cells_

6. Hypothermia *condition of less heat*

7. Mononucleosis *condition of one central structure*

8. Decimeter *instrument to record 1000*

9. Diplopia *double vision*

10. Triorchidism *condition of 3 testis*

11. Pantophobia *fear of all*

12. Unilateral *one sided*

13. Oligodontia *condition of less teeth*

14. Hyperglycosuria *condition of more sugar in urine*

Section D

Construct terms for the following.

1. Many blood cells *polysomatocyte*

2. Removal of half a lung *pleo*

3. Condition of more color _____

4. Little urine _____

5. Deficiency of all (blood) cells _____

6. Pertaining to many joints _____

7. Paralysis of one muscle _____

8. Pertaining to one sex _____

9. Having three cusps _____

10. One hundred liters _____

11. Pertaining to two ears _____

12. Two-color vision _____

13. Resembling single (set of chromosomes) _____

14. Little menstrual flow _____

15. Having four sides _____

16. Four monosaccharides _____

17. Pertaining to less cholesterol in blood _____

18. More bilirubin in the blood _____

19. One-hundredth of a liter _____

20. Inflammation of all (parts) of a bone _____

TERMINOLOGY SEARCH 6: DIAGNOSIS CHECKLIST

Reproduced here is a diagnosis checklist used by a medical center. The conditions were selected from the International Classification of Diseases, ninth revision, Clinical Modification (ICD-9-CM), which is prepared by the World Health Organization. The numerical codes are used by medical insurers.

DIAGNOSIS

CARDIOLOGY

413.9	Angina Pectoris
4402	Arteriosclerosis, Extremities
4229	Arteriosclerotic Heart Disease
4274	Atrial Fibrillation
4279	Cardiac Arrhythmia
786.50	Chest Pain
7469	Congential Heart Defect
4270	Congestive Heart Failure
7823	Edema
4269	Heart Block and/or Strokes Adams Syndrome
4011	Hypertension
4020	Hypertensive Heart Disease
4580	Hypotension, Orthostatic
4109	Myocardial Infarction, Acute
4107	Myocardial Infarction. Convalescent
7851	Palpitations
4439	Peripheral Vascular Disease
4519	Phlebitis and Thrombophlebitis
7850	Tachycardia
4247	Valvular Disease (Non-Rheumatic)
3979	Valvular Disease (Rheumatic)
4549	Varicose Veins

DERMATOLOGY

Code	Diagnosis
7061	Acne
6809	Carbuncle, Furuncle, Boil
6929	Dermatitis, Nonspecific
6929	Eczema, Nonspecific
1119	Fungal Dermatitis
0539	Herpes Zoster
6840	Impetigo
6958	Intertrigo, Monilial
6989	Pruritis
7089	Urticaria
6923	Allergic-dermatitis
7063	Seborrhea

EENT

372.30	Conjunctivitis
7847	Epistaxis
3659	Glaucoma
7844	Hoarseness, Etiology Undeter
3863	Labyrinthitis
4640	Laryngitis/Tracheitis, Acute
3801	Otitis Externa
3829	Otitis Media
3810	Otitis Serous
462	Pharyngitis, Acute
4779	Rhinitis, Allergic
4610	Sinusitis
5280	Stomatitis
463	Tonsillitis, Acute

ENDOCRINOLOGY

Code	Diagnosis
250.00	Diabetes Mellitus
2409	Goiter
2720	Hypercholesterolemia
2754	Hypercalcemia
7906	Hyperglycemia
2724	Hyperlipemia
2429	Hyperthroidism
2721	Hypertriglyceridemia
7906	Hyperuricemia
2449	Hypothyroidism
7832	Loss of Weight
2639	Malnutrition
2770	Obesity
2419	Thyroid Nodule
6270	Menopausal Symptoms
2512	Hypoglycemia

GASTROENTEROLOGY

Code	Diagnosis
7893	Abdominal Mass
7890	Abdominal Pain/Colic
5300	Achalasia
5650	Anal Fissure
7830	Anorexia
5400	Appendicitis
7895	Ascites
5300	Chalasia
5751	Cholecystitis
5744	Cholelithiasis
5715	Cirrhosis
5559	Crohn's Disease
5640	Constipation
5589	Diarrhea
5305	Diffuse Esophageal Spasm
5620	Diverticulitis
56211	Diverticulosis, Colon
7872	Dysphagia
5301	Esophagitis
5649	Functional Intestinal Disorder
5350	Gastritis/Duodenitis
5889	Gastroenteritis/Colitis-Acute
5789	G. I. Bleeding
7871	Heartburn
5780	Hematemesis
4556	Hemorrhoids
0701	Hepatitis-Infectious
5733	Hepatitis-Chronic Active
7891	Hepatomegaly
5513	Hernia-Hiatal
5500	Hernia-Other
5609	Intestinal Obstruction
5641	Irritable Colon/Bowel
7852	Jaundice
5781	Melena
7870	Nausea/Vomiting
5770	Pancreatitis
566	Perirectal Absess
6851	Pilonidal Cyst
5319	Ulcer-Gastric
53390	Ulcer Peptic
5560	Ulcerative Colitis

GYNECOLOGY

Code	Diagnosis
6202	Cyst, Ovarian
6160	Chronic-Cervicitis
2540	Contraception
6469	Complication of Pregnancy
V2541	Pill
V2542	IUD
6101	Cystic Disease of Breast Chronic
61172	Breast Mass
6159	Endometriosis
V222	Pregnancy
6149	Pelvic Inflamation Disease
6273	Vaginitis, Atrophic
61610	Vaginitis, Non-Specific
13101	Vaginitis, Trichomonal
1121	Vaginitis, Monilial
6260	Amenorrhea
6262	Menometrorrhagia
6259	Pelvic Pain

HEMATOLOGY

2809	Anemia-Iron Deficient
2859	Anemia Nonspecific
2800	Anemia-Due To Blood Loss
2810	Anemia-Pernicious
28260	Anemia-Sickle Cell
2387	Myeloproliferative disease
2839	Anemia-hemolytic

INFECTIOUS & PARASITIC DISEASE

566	Absess-Perirectal
6829	Absess-Subcutaneous
0049	Bacillary Enteritis
6822	Cellulitis
0529	Chicken Pox
4644	Croup
460	Common Cold
3229	Meningitis
0059	Food Poisoning
0980	Gonococcal Infection
684	Impetigo
075	Infectious Mononucleosis
4871	Influenza
1121	Monillasis
6819	Paronychia
1329	Pediculosis
0979	Syphilis
1310	Trichomoniasis, Urogenital
0119	Tuberculosis
2893	Viral Infection-Lymphadenitis
78609	URI
5990	UTI

MISCELLANEOUS

Code	Diagnosis
7870	Nausea/Vomiting
9952	Allergy-Drug
7999	Diagnosis Unknown-Deferred
7804	Dizziness
7834	Failure to Thrive
7806	Fever-Unknown Origin
72743	Ganglion Cyst
9999	General Exam, No Disease
7807	Malaise
6851	Pilonidal Cyst
2780	Obesity
7802	Syncope
7373	Scoliosis
7807	Weakness/Fatigue
V202	Well Child
7832	Weight Loss

GENITOURINARY

5920	Calculus-Renal or Ureteral
5959	Cystitis
7883	Enuresis
5839	Glomerulonephritis
5997	Hematuria
60784	Impotence
7910	Proteinuria
6000	Prostatic Hypertrophy Benign
6019	Prostatitis
5908	Pyelonephritis
5939	Renal Insufficiency
5978	Urethritis
5990	Urinary Tract Infection
6039	Hydrocoele

NEUROLOGY & PSYCHIATRY

3039	Alcoholism
7813	Ataxia
3000	Anxiety
4350	Basilar Artery Insufficiency
4292	Cerebrovascular Accident
3109	Chronic Brain Syndrome
2900	Dementia-Senile
311	Depression
7804	Dizziness
7840	Headache
3469	Headache-Migraine
78601	Hyperventilation Syndrome
78052	Insomnia
3152	Learning Disability
7992	Nervousness
7820	Numbness
3320	Parkinson's Disease
3579	Peripheral Nueropathy
3160	Psychogenic Disorder
2919	Psychosis-Alcoholic
3099	Situation Adj. Reaction
7803	Seizures
4359	Transient Cerebral Ischemia
7804	Vertigo

ONCOLOGY

Code	Diagnosis
1991	Malignant Neoplasm
2299	Benign Neoplasm
2399	Unspecified Neoplasm

PULMONARY DISEASE

Code	Diagnosis
4939	Asthma
490.0	Bronchitis
4660	Bronchiolitis-Acute
7862	Cough
78609	Dyspnea
5109	Emphysema
496	Obstructive Lung Disease, Chronic
4829	Pneumonia-Bacterial
4809	Pneumonia-Viral
4151	Pulmonary Embolism or Infarction
5150	Pulmonary Fibrosis
135	Sarcoidosis
0119	Tuberculosis

RHEUMATOLOGY

Code	Diagnosis
7273	Bursitis-Synovitis
3540	Carpal Tunnel Syndrome
7159	Degenerative Arthritis
7295	Extremity Pain
2749	Gout
71940	Joint Pain
7242	Low Back Pain
6954	Lupus Erythematosus
8460	Lumbosacral Sprain
7288	Muscle Spasm
7291	Myalgia
7159	Osteoarthritis
7330	Osteoporosis
7140	Rheumatoid Arthritis-Adult
7143	Rheumatoid Arthritis-Juvenile
7243	Sciatica
7269	Tendonitis

TRAUMA

9190	Abrasion
9490	Burn
8509	Concussion
9249	Contusion
8398	Dislocation w/o FX
9309	Foreign Body-Ear
932	Foreign Bcdy-Nose
9350	Foreign Body-Mouth
810.00	Fracture-Upper Limb
82382	Fracture-Lower Limb
8248	Fracture-Ankle
807.00	Fracture-Rib
9224	Hematoma
8798	Laceration
988.0	Food Poisoning
8798	Puncture Wound
8489	Sprain/Strain

Diagnosis (Not Listed):

_____

_____

_____

Furnished by Memorial Medical Clinic, Richmond, Virginia.

A Potpourri of Sources 1
Words From Languages Other Than Greek and Latin

Potpourri: from French, meaning hotchpotch (stew); from the words for shake and pot, therefore a collection of different kinds

Almost all the word elements you have learned thus far are from either Greek or Latin. Our linguistic[1] heritage, however, has been enriched by contributions from a number of other languages. The purpose of this lesson is to give you a sampling from this source. Some explanatory notes are included for your interest.

Term	Usage	Original Meaning or Explanatory Notes
German		
mittelschmerz	ovulation pain	middle pain
ketone	chemical produced in metabolism	from acetone
French		
cretin	person with congenital hypothyroidism	
fontanelles	soft spots in infant's skull	little fountain
tourniquet	instrument to prevent loss of blood	turning instrument
venom	poison injected by animal or insect bite or sting	poison
cul de sac	a blind-end area	bottom of the sack
chancre	symptom of primary syphilis	ulcer

[1] Note the use of the root lingua, tongue, in a different sense here.

177

Term	Usage	Original Meaning or Explanatory Notes
French		
goiter	hyperplasia of thyroid	from word for throat
malaise	discomfort, unease	bad ease
douche	current of water or vapor	shower
massage	pressure and friction on the skin	knead
morgue	repository for corpses	stare at
calorie	measure of energy	heat
tampon	material to absorb body secretions	plug
Italian		
belladonna	drug used to dilate pupils	beautiful lady
influenza	viral infection	flow in
malaria	protozoan infection (proto = first) (zoo = animal)	bad air
Arabic		
camphor	topical antipruritic (prur = itching)	
alcohol		something subtle
elixir	alcoholic solution	philosopher's stone
bezoar	stone from animal stomach	protection against poison; antidote (given against)
caffeine	stimulant	
arsenic	ingredient of dyes and medicines	ointment
senna	a purgative	

178

Term	Usage	Original Meaning or Explanatory Notes
East Indian		
kala-azar	a protozoan infection	black fever
beriberi	deficiency of thiamine (one of of the B vitamin complex)	great weakness
South American Indian		
curare	muscle relaxant	
quinine	antimalarial drug	
ipecac	an emetic	low leaves and roots
African		
kwashiorkor	protein deficiency	red or golden boy
tsetse	fly transmitting protozoan sleeping sickness	
Spanish		
cascara sagrada	a laxative	sacred bark
marijuana	intoxicating drug with possible medical uses	Mary Jane
Dutch		
cough	violent, forceful expiration	
splint	appliance to fix a body part in place	wedge

Term	Usage	Original Meaning or Explanatory Notes
	Persian	
borax	detergent; weak antiseptic	
talc	dusting powder	

There are no practice exercises with this lesson. Begin working on Review Test 2, which starts on page 185.

A Potpourri of Sources 2
Words From Mythology, Word Transformation, Coined Words, Drug Names, Trade Names

---

Potpourri: from French, meaning hotchpotch (stew); from the words for shake and pot, therefore a collection of different kinds

---

1. Greek and Roman mythology is a natural source of terms that have been handed down to us through the languages of these cultures. Following are a few such terms.

    Achilles' tendon: tendon attaching to the calcaneus (heel bone).

    > Achilles' mother dipped him in the River Styx to confer immortality upon him. She held him by the heel, rendering him vulnerable there where the water did not touch him.

    Arachnoid: resembling a spider web

    > Arachne was a peasant girl with great skill in weaving who was changed into a spider by the jealous goddess Minerva.

    Hermaphroditic: having both sexes

    > Hermes was the messenger of Zeus; Aphrodite was the goddess of love and beauty. Note also that an aphrodisiac is a drug that stimulates sexual desire.

    Hippocampus: a part of the cerebrum shaped like a seahorse

    > The gods rode on a seahorse, hence this name (hippos = horse; campus = sea monster).

    Hygiene

    > This term comes from Hygeia, the Greek goddess of health.

    Hymen: a membrane partially closing the vaginal opening

    > Hymen was the god of the wedding feast.

    Iris: the colored ring in the eye

    > Iris was the goddess of the rainbow.

    Labyrinth: a complex structure of the inner ear

    > Labyrinth was the name of a maze in which was kept the minotaur, a creature who was half man, half bull.

    Panacea: a cure-all

    > Panacea was the Greek goddess of healing.

Psyche: mind (originally soul)

    Psyche was a princess who married Cupid, the God of Love.

Syphilis: a venereal disease (see next entry)

    This is the title of a sixteenth-century poem concerning Syphilus, a shepherd who had a sexually transmitted disease and bathed in a sea of mercury.

Venereal: disease transmitted by sexual contact

    Venereal is the adjective form of Venus, the Roman goddess of love and beauty, the equivalent to the Greek Aphrodite.

2. Some terms have originated through variations in pronunciation or spelling or both over a period of time. It is interesting to trace such terms to their sources.

Term	Meaning	Derivation
migraine	severe headache	from hemicranial
rickets	malformation of bone due to vitamin D deficiency	from rachitis
shingles	virus infection of nerve endings	from cingulum = girdle
palsy	lack of muscle coordination	from paralysis
frenzy	hyperagitation	from phrenitis
surgery		from chirurgy = handwork
pleurisy	inflammation of the membrane of the lungs	from pleuritis

3. You will run across medical terms that have been coined to fit particular situations. For example:

Term	Meaning	Derivation
endorphin	chemical secreted in brain that alleviates pain	shortening of *endogenous morphine*
lumpectomy	removal of a lump in the breast	
oncornavirus	RNA virus that causes tumors	
dosimetry	measurement of doses	
interferon	produced in the body during virus infection	interferes with virus reproduction
warfarin	antithrombotic drug	from the initials of the *Wisconsin Alumni Research Foundation* and cou*marin* (anticoagulant chemical)
prostaglandins	group of hormones present in many tissues	first ones in group discovered in prostate gland

4. A discussion of the derivation of names of drugs is beyond the scope of this book. Drug names are derived from many and varied sources. Some of these names are obvious, as in the following generic names:

    Sulfa drugs contain sulfur.

    Penicillin comes from the genus of the mold that produces it, *Penicillium*.

Other generic names with interesting histories include:

    Digitalis, a heart-regulating drug, is made by a plant that bears leaves in an arrangement resembling fingers (digits).

Aspirin is derived from the chemical name of the compound, which is acetyl salicylic acid. The a of aspirin is from acetyl, and the spir is from spirsaure, another name for salicylic acid. (Salicylic acid was discovered in the willow tree, which has the genus name *Salix*.)

As you encounter trade names of drugs, see whether you can determine their sources. For example:

Coricidin means literally "kill a cold" (cor- from Greek coryza = nasal discharge).

Robitussin is a cough medicine made by A. H. Robins Co.; robi- from the company name, -tuss = cough (pertussis, whooping cough = violent cough).

5. Finally, consider a sampling of the trade names of products related to oral hygiene.

Lavoris = mouthwash

Dentyne = teeth

Polident = many teeth

Pepsodent = digest teeth

There are no practice exercises for this lesson. Continue your review by working on Review Test 2.

Review Test 2

Suggestions for using this material:

Go through and write the answers you are sure of.

Review the word elements and their meanings in Lessons 13 through 22.

Record additional answers that you have recalled by this method.

Look up any items remaining and record your answers. You may want to review Lessons 3 through 12 at this point.

Check your answers with the key.

Cover your answers with a sheet of paper and take the test again.

Additional or alternative review methods:

Work through the practice exercises with each lesson.

Read through the Glossary-Index of Word Elements, which includes all word elements in the book.

Examine the labels on the illustrations throughout the book. You should now be able to appreciate the logical nature of the nomenclature of body parts.

Review the Terminology Search exercises.

Note: Be sure to work on the frequently confused word elements listed at the end of this review test.

Section A

Following are a few of the multitude of terms that are necessary in learning human anatomy. Define each to the extent that you can; some extra words are included to indicate the type of structure described.

1. Corpora cavernosa _____

2. Pulmonary hilum _____

3. Brachial plexus _____

4. Sarcolemma _____

5. Greater tubercle of the humerus _____

6. External auditory meatus _____

7. Gastric fundus _____

8. Septum lucidum _____

9. Ischial ramus _____

10. Tensor fasciae latae muscle _____ _____

11. Hypoglossal nerve _____

12. Pharyngotympanic tube _____

13. Internal nares _____

14. Parathyroid _____

15. Pyloric sphincter _____

16. Renal papilla _____

17. Seminiferous tubule _____

18. Epiglottis _____

19. Visceral pleura _____

20. Phrenic artery _____

21. Adenohypophysis _____

22. Neuroglia _____

23. Sudoriferous glands _____

24. Vitreous humor _____

25. Cytoplasm _____

26. Sebaceous gland _____

27. Myometrium _____

28. Mamillary bodies (in brain) _____

29. Choroid layer of eyeball _____

30. Perirenal adipose tissue _____

31. Anterior cranial fossa _____

32. Insular lobe of cerebrum _____

33. Venous lumen _____

34. Cystic rugae _____

35. Striated muscle _____

36. Pilomotor muscle _____

37. Posterior primary ramus of spinal nerve _____

38. Reticular tissue _____

39. Lingual tonsil _____

40. Mesentery _____

41. Stratum corneum of epidermis _____

42. Optic chiasma _____

43. Bone lamellae _____

44. Perimysium _____

45. Nasopharynx _____

46. Collagenous fibers _____

47. Hyaline cartilage _____

48. Seminal vesicle _____

49. Platysma muscle _____

50. Gastrocnemius muscle _____

51. Semitendinosus muscle _____

52. Tunica media of blood vessel wall _____

Section B

Following are a few of the terms used in human physiology. Derive meanings to the extent that you have learned them.

1. Metabolism _____

2. Amylase _____

3. Glucose _____

4. Lysosome _____

5. Hemostasis _____

6. Alveolar air _____

7. Adrenocorticotropin _____

8. Polysaccharide _____

9. Isotonic saline _____

10. Acromegaly _____

11. Lactogenic hormone _____

12. Meiosis _____

13. Corpus luteum _____

14. Gametogenesis _____

15. Epinephrine _____

16. Myxedema _____

17. Gonadotropin _____

18. Phagocytosis _____

19. Hemolysis _____

20. Progesterone _____

21. Nucleoli _____

Section C

Analyze the following medical terms by dividing them into their elements. Then give the definition.

1. Dyscrasia _____

2. Diagnostic _____

3. Allergy _____

4. Hypertrophy _____

5. Gastroclysis _____

6. Laparorrhaphy _____

7. Podiatrist _____

8. Myomectomy _____

9. Biliary stasis _____

10. Hidradenitis _____

11. Oliguria _____

12. *Saccharomyces* (genus of yeast) _____

13. Mucocolitis _____

14. Pharmacopeia (simplified spelling of -poieia), an authoritative book _____

15. Sialophagia _____

16. Transurethral prostatectomy _____

17. Hysterodynia _____

18. Baryphonia _____

19. Cyanotic _____

20. Megalomania _____

21. Hepatocirrhosis _____

22. Anosmia _____

23. Streptococcal _____

24. Pantophobia _____

25. Pleocytosis _____

26. Electrophoresis _____

27. Cacodontia _____

28. Prophylaxis _____

29. Phalangotripsy _____

30. Bronchiolitis _____

Section D

Construct medical terms for the following definitions. Words in parentheses are for explanation only.

1. Recording of color _____

2. Study of cause _____

3. False pregnancy _____

4. Inflammation of gall bladder _____

5. Flow of pus _____

6. Herniation of esophagus _____

7. Puncture of amnion _____

8. Removal of half of a lung _____

9. Spasm of the diaphragm _____

10. More than normal pituitary (secretion) _____

11. Softening of cartilage _____

12. Less than normal sodium in the blood _____

13. Gallstones _____

14. Pain in many muscles _____

15. Instrument to examine the vagina _____

16. Fungous conditions of the lungs _____

17. Poison in the blood _____

18. Dry skin _____

19. Gray tumor _____

20. Broad, flat nails _____

21. Tumor of smooth muscle _____

22. Pertaining to two colors _____

23. Split mind _____

24. Pertaining to the healing of children _____

FREQUENTLY CONFUSED WORD ELEMENTS

Experience has shown that the following word elements are frequently confused. If you are not sure of the meanings, look them up and record them here. A careful study of this list will help you avoid making errors in deriving word meanings. Test yourself by covering your written definitions.

adeno/adreno _____ / _____

algesia/esthesia _____ / _____

ante/anti _____ / _____

aero/acro _____ / _____

brachy/brachi _____ / _____

brachy/brady _____ / _____

brachy/trachy _____ / _____

cyto/cysto _____ / _____

ectopy/ectomy _____ / _____

ectopy/ectasia _____ / _____

edema/emia _____ / _____

emesis/emia _____ / _____

hidro/hydro _____ / _____

hydro/hygro _____ / _____

hepato/hemato _____ / _____

hemi/hemo _____ / _____

ileum/ilium _____ / _____

lysis/clysis _____ / _____

lacri/lacto _____ / _____

myo/myxo _____ / _____

myxo/myco _____ / _____

myo/myco _____ / _____

myo/myelo _____ / _____

melano/megalo _____ / _____

melano/malacia _____ / _____

oral/oval _____ / _____

pyo/pyro _____ / _____

pyelo/myelo _____ / _____

phasia/phagia _____ / _____

psycho/psychro _____ / _____

stoma/soma _____ / _____

striat/strati _____ / _____

stenosis/centesis _____ / _____

spino/spiro _____ / _____

tachy/trachy _____ / _____

top/trop _____ / _____

trop/troph _____ / _____

uretero/urethro _____ / _____

uretero/utero _____ / _____

veni/vesico _____ / _____

Answers to Review Test 2—page 240

P.S.

Post scripto: From Latin, meaning written after

If you have worked carefully through this book you now have a vocabulary of about 550 word elements that are used to build terms referring to the human body and medical conditions and procedures. You have only begun, however. In the future you will encounter many other terms in textbooks and in reading newspapers and magazines. Keep a medical dictionary handy and look up new terms as you encounter them. Record new words below for handy reference. The more you do this, the easier future learning will be for you in a health science profession. If you get rusty, work through the book again.

Word Element	**Meaning**
_____	_____
_____	_____
_____	_____
_____	_____
_____	_____
_____	_____
_____	_____
_____	_____
_____	_____
_____	_____
_____	_____
_____	_____
_____	_____
_____	_____
_____	_____
_____	_____
_____	_____

Word Element	Meaning

Greek and Latin

More than three-fourths of today's medical vocabulary has been derived from Greek and Latin. New words are coined largely from Greek. These languages have been important not just in medical terminology but in the development of the English language generally. More than 50% of the most common English words owe their origin to Greek and Latin. All three languages belong to the Indo-European group, as do French, Spanish, Italian, German, and most of the other modern European tongues.

As you might guess, the story of the interweaving influences that have worked through the years on language development is a complex one. Suffice it to say that you can recognize the elements you have learned in this book in many of the words that are a part of your general vocabulary. To the degree that you are on the lookout for them, your comprehension of the English language will be strengthened. This appendix describes a few of the basics of Greek and Latin that should aid you in your understanding. Perhaps you will be interested enough to take a course in one or both of them.

LATIN

The Latin alphabet is like the English, except that there is no j or w. Due to this similarity, most of the Latin terms, many of which were transliterated from Greek, resemble the English forms that we use.

Note: The letter i used as a consonant in Latin comes into English as a j.

maior ⟶ major

GREEK

In studying Greek as a language, you must first learn a different alphabet (from alpha and beta, the first two letters). Following is a listing of the Greek alphabet and the English equivalents. Only the small letters are given. You may encounter some Greek letters in medical terminology.

alpha	α	a
beta	β	b
gamma	γ	g
delta	δ	d
epsilon	ϵ	e
zeta	ζ	z
eta	η	e
theta	θ	th
iota	ι	i
kappa	κ	k or c
lambda	λ	l
mu	μ	m
nu	ν	n
xi	ξ	x

omicron	*o*	o
pi	π	p
rho	ρ	r
sigma	ς when final letter; otherwise ϭ	s
tau	τ	t
upsilon	υ	y (u in diphthongs)
phi	φ	ph or f
chi	χ	ch
psi	ψ	ps
omega	ω	o

1. There are two Greek letters that transliterate into English as e and two that become o.

2. The Greek gamma changes to an n in English before certain consonants.

$$γαγγλιον \rightarrow \text{ganglion}$$

3. The Greek k often is changed to c in English, but with a hard pronunciation.

$$λευκος \rightarrow \text{leuco-}$$

4. The sound of the English h is achieved in Greek only at the beginning of a word by a "rough breathing" mark ('). This mark comes into English as h. The h is placed preceding a beginning vowel, but following a beginning rho. In addition, the rho often is doubled when it occurs in the middle of a word in English.

$$αἷμα \rightarrow \text{hema-}$$
$$ῥειν \rightarrow \text{-rrhea}$$

5. There is no Greek equivalent for the English j, q, v, or w.

BOTH GREEK AND LATIN

1. The singular and plural endings of medical words in English are often those used in Greek or Latin.

Singular	Plural
stoma	stomata
fungus	fungi
phalanx	phalanges

2. In many cases, the word roots that we use to build terms come from forms that appear in the inflection of Greek and Latin words. (Inflection refers to changes in spelling to indicate changes in function; for example, declension of nouns or adjectives and conjugation of verbs.)

$$πους \rightarrow \text{pous} = \text{foot}$$

Another form is podos (pod-).

pulmo = Lung

Another form is pulmonis (pulmon-).

stare = to stand

Another form is statum (stat-).

$$λαβειν \rightarrow \text{labein} = \text{to seize}$$

Another form is lep- (-lepsy).

3. Greek and Latin diphthongs (from Greek, meaning two sounds) usually are simplified in English to single vowels.

caecum → cecum

Χειρ = cheir ⟶ chir = hand

4. Some medical terms are hybrid; that is, they use roots from both languages.

append/ectomy   hyper/tension

Latin   Greek   Greek   Latin

Abbreviations

These abbreviations are illustrative of a large number in use in a number of medical disciplines. Most of them can be found in medical dictionaries; some are popular or medical lingo (from Latin; lingua = tongue).

a.c.	before meals (L. ante cibum)
ACTH	adrenocorticotropic hormone
ADH	antidiuretic hormone
ad lib.	as desired (L. ad libitum)
ANS	autonomic nervous system
A & P	auscultation and percussion
APC	aspirin, phenacetin, caffeine
Aq.	water (L. aqua)
ARD	acute respiratory distress
AV	atrioventricular; arteriovenous
Av.	average; avoirdupois weight
BBT	basal body temperature
b.i.d.	twice a day (L. bis in die)
BM	bowel movement
B.M.R.	basal metabolic rate
B.P.	blood pressure
B.S.	blood sugar; breath sounds
BSA	body surface area
BT	bleeding time
BUN	blood urea nitrogen
C.	Celsius
c	with (L. cum)
Ca	cancer
ca.	about (L. circa)
CAT scan	computerized axial tomography
c.b.c.	complete blood count
cc	cubic centimeter
CCU	coronary care unit
CHD	coronary heart disease
CHF	congestive heart failure

cm	centimeter
CMV	cytomegalovirus
C.N.S.	central nervous system
COPD	chronic obstructive pulmonary disease
CPR	cardiopulmonary resuscitation
C-section	cesarean section
C.S.F.	cerebrospinal fluid
CST	convulsive shock therapy
CVA	cerebrovascular accident
CVS	cardiovascular system
D & C	dilatation and curettage
D.D.S.	Doctor of Dental Surgery
D.O.A.	dead on arrival
DPT	diphtheria, pertussis, tetanus
dx	diagnosis
ECG	electrocardiogram
E.D.	effective dose
EEG	electroencephalogram
EKG	electrocardiogram
E.N.T.	ear, nose, throat
ESP	extrasensory perception
E.S.T.	electroshock therapy
F.	Fahrenheit
FBS	fasting blood sugar
FH	family history
Fl.	fluid
FSH	follicle-stimulating hormone
F.U.O.	fever of undetermined origin
fx	fracture
GB	gall bladder
G.I.	gastrointestinal
gm	gram
G.P.	general practitioner
GTH	gonadotropic hormone
GU	genitourinary
GYN	gynecology
Hb	hemoglobin
HCG	human chorionic gonadotropin

HCT	hematocrit
HGH	human growth hormone
h.s.	at bedtime (L. hora somni)
HVD	hypertensive vascular disease
hypo	hypodermic
ICU	intensive care unit
ID	intradermal
I & D	incision and drainage
Ig	immunoglobulin
I.H.	infectious hepatitis
I.M.	intramuscular
I.P.	intraperitoneal
IUD	intrauterine device
I.V.	intravenous
kg	kilogram
K.U.B.	kidney, ureter, bladder
LD	lethal dose
LGH	lactogenic hormone
LH	luteinizing hormone
L.M.P.	last menstrual period
LP	lumbar puncture
L.P.N.	Licensed Practical Nurse
M.D.	Doctor of Medicine
M.E.D.	minimal effective dose
mg	milligram
MI	myocardial infarction
ml	milliliter
M.M.	mucous membrane
mm	millimeter
MS	multiple sclerosis
N.A.D.	no appreciable disease
NG	nasogastric
NPN	nonprotein nitrogen
NPO	nothing by mouth (L. nihil per os)
N.T.P.	normal temperature and pressure
OB	obstetrics
OD	overdose
O.R.	operating room

OT	occupational therapy
OTC	over the counter
P.A.	Physician's Assistant
Pap test	Papanicolaou's test
PAT	paroxysmal atrial tachycardia
PBI	protein-bound iodine
p.c.	after meals (L. post cibum)
PCG	phonocardiogram
PCV	packed cell volume
P.D.R.	Physician's Desk Reference
PEG	pneumoencephalogram
pH	hydrogen ion concentration
P.I.D.	pelvic inflammatory disease
PKU	phenylketonuria
P.M.	post mortem
P.O.	by mouth (L. per os); postoperative
poly	polymorphonuclear leukocyte
p.r.n.	as need arises (L. pro re nata)
PT	physical therapy
pt.	patient
PVC	premature ventricular contraction
q.d.	every day (L. quaque die)
q.h.	every hour (L. quaque hora)
q.i.d.	four times a day (L. quater in die)
q.l.	as much as desired (L. quantum libet)
q.s.	sufficient (L. quantum satis)
rad	radiation unit
R.B.C.	red blood cell; red blood count
REM	rapid eye movement
Rep.	repeat
Rh	Rhesus factor
R.N.	Registered Nurse
R/O	rule out
Rx	take (L. recipe)
s	without (L. sine)
S.D.	skin dose
Sig.	let it be labeled (L. signetur)
SLE	systemic lupus erythematosus
SOB	shortness of breath

sp. gr.	specific gravity
SQ	subcutaneous
S.R.	sedimentation rate
St.	let it stand (L. stet)
stat.	immediately (L. statim)
S.T.S.	serological test for syphilis
T.A.	toxin-antitoxin
TB	tuberculosis
TBI	total body irradiation
t.i.d.	three times a day (L. ter in die)
TLC	total lung capacity; tender loving care
TPR	temperature, pulse, respiration
TSA	tumor specific antigen
TSH	thyroid-stimulating hormone
tus.	cough (L. tussis)
U.	unit
URI	upper respiratory infection
U.S.P.	United States Pharmacopeia
ut dict.	as directed (L. ut dictum)
VC	vital capacity
V.D.	venereal disease
V.D.H.	valvular disease of the heart
W.B.C.	white blood cell; white blood count
WD	well-developed
WN	well-nourished
wt.	weight

References

Agard, W. G., and H.M. Rowe. 1955. *Medical Greek and Latin at a Glance*, 3d ed. New York: Harper and Row.

Asimov, I. 1969. *Words of Science*. New York: New American Library (Mentor).

Borror, D. J. 1960. *Dictionary of Word Roots and Combining Forms*. Palo Alto: Mayfield.

Cole, F. 1970. *The Doctor's Shorthand*. Philadelphia: Saunders.

Dirckx, J. H. 1976. *The Language of Medicine*. Hagerstown, Maryland: Harper and Row (Medical Department).

Dorland's Illustrated Medical Dictionary, 26th ed. 1981. Philadelphia: Saunders.

Gray, P. 1973. *Student Dictionary of Biology*. New York: Van Nostrand/Reinhold.

Jaeger, E.C. 1953. *A Sourcebook of Medical Terms*. Springfield, Illinois: Charles C. Thomas.

Knight, B. 1980. *Discovering the Human Body*. New York: Lippincott and Crowell.

The Medical and Health Sciences Wordbook. 1977. Boston: Houghton-Mifflin.

Nybakken, O. E. 1959. *Greek and Latin in Scientific Terminology*. Ames: Iowa State University Press.

Prichard, R.W., and R. E. Robinson. 1972. *Twenty Thousand Medical Words*. New York: McGraw-Hill.

Sloane, S. B. 1973. *The Medical Word Book: A Spelling and Pronunciation Guide to Medical Transcription*. Philadelphia: Saunders.

Smith, R. W. C. 1966. *Dictionary of English Word Roots*. Totowa, New Jersey: Littlefield, Adams and Co.

Stegeman, W. 1976. *Medical Terms Simplified*. St. Paul: West.

Willeford, G. 1976. *Medical Word Finder*, 2d ed. Englewood Cliffs, New Jersey: Prentice-Hall.

Answer Key

LESSON 1

therm o graph ic
WR CV WR S
  CF

dys men o rrhea
P WR CV S
    CF

cyst o scopy
WR CV S
  CF

phleb ectas ia
WR   WR S

pro gnosis
P WR

lapar o tomy
WR CV S
  CF

blephar o plasty
WR CV S
  CF

ather o scler osis
WR CV WR S
  CF

hepat itis
WR S

col o stomy
WR CV S
  CF

syn chondr osis
P WR S

hem o phil ia
WR CV WR S
  CF

carcin o gen ic
WR CV WR S
  CF

angi o gram
WR CV S
  CF

an esthes ia
P WR S

hemi pleg ic
P WR S

nephr o lith
WR CV S
  CF

bin ocul ar
P WR S

oste o por osis
WR CV WR S
  CF

electr o cardi o gram
WR CV WR CV S
  CF   CF

LESSON 2

1. Hypodermic
2. Dysentery
3. Anemia
4. Dermatology
5. Mastectomy
6. Dermatitis
7. Hepatosis
8. Pericardial
9. Posthepatic
10. Cardiogram
11. Anencephaly
12. Enteric
13. Hematology
14. Endoscope
15. Mastitis
16. Endocarditis
17. Thermogram
18. Encephalitis
19. Perimastic
20. Hypocardiac
21. Postenterectomy
22. Amastia
23. Endohepatic
24. Hypothermia
25. Dyshepatia

LESSON 3

Section A

1. Cervico-
2. Axilla
3. Auriculo-
4. Plantar
5. Dactylo-
6. Parieto-
7. Carpo-
8. Brachio-
9. Femoro-
10. Thoraco-

Section B

1. Antebrachium
2. Onycho-
3. Tarso-
4. Inguino-
5. Mento-
6. Olecrano-
7. Coxo-
8. Cnemo-
9. Laparo-
10. Carpo-

208

Section C

1. Eye   oculo-
2. Navel   omphalo-
3. Lip   labio-
4. Head   cephalo-
5. Viscera   viscero-
6. Skin   cutaneo-

   integumento-
7. Foot   podo-
8. Chest   stetho-
9. Breast   mammo-
10. Nose   naso-

Section D

1. Bucco-
2. Abdomino-
3. Lumbo-
4. Chiro-
5. Thel-

6. Brachio-
7. Gluteo-
8. Genu-
9. Popliteal
10. Plantar

Section E

1. Pain in the head
2. Specialist in study of the eyes
3. Instrument to examine the chest
4. Incision into the abdominal wall
5. More than normal digits

6. Large (muscle) of the chest
7. Inflammation of the navel
8. Pertaining to the cheek
9. Pertaining to two eyes
10. Pertaining to the breast

Section F

1. Mastectomy
2. ~~Lumbar~~ ≠ groin (loin)
3. Abdominocentesis
4. Subcutaneous
5. Onychophagia

6. Podiatrist
7. Cheiloplasty
8. Splanchomegaly, visceromegaly
9. Dermopathy
10. Celiac

LESSON 4

Section A

Suffix	Example
1. -ectomy	appendectomy
2. -itis	tonsillitis
3. -oid	colloid
4. -scopy	microscopy
5. -clast	osteoclast
6. -ic, -al	hepatic, dermal
7. -genesis	spermatogenesis
8. -logy	psychology
9. -osis, -ia	nephrosis, hypothermia
10. -meter	barometer

Section B

Suffix	Example
1. -gram	cardiogram
2. -lysis	hemolysis
3. -penia	cytopenia
4. -stomy	tracheostomy
5. -tomy	thoracotomy
6. -megaly	splenomegaly
7. -rrhea	diarrhea
8. -stenosis	vasostenosis
9. -ist	dentist
10. -ectasia	bronchiectasia

Section C

1. -genesis, -plasia, -poiesis
2. -ic, -al, -ary, -ous, -ar, -eal, -ory, -iac
3. -ia, -y, -osis, -iasis, -ism
4. -ia, -y

Note: Often in writing definitions the words "pertaining to," "condition," and "process" are omitted. We will do so later in the book. For now, keep these meanings in mind to help you understand word construction.

Section D

1. Enzyme

2. Full of, carbohydrate

3. Break down

4. Instrument to record

5. Specialist in the study of

6. Instrument to examine

7. Crushing, friction

Section E

1.	Mast/oid	resembling a breast
2.	Steth/o/scope	instrument to examine the chest
3.	Rhin/itis	inflammation of the nose
4.	Mamm/o/gram	record of the breast
5.	Lapar/o/tomy	incision into the abdominal wall
6.	Ophthalm/o/logy	study of the eyes
7.	Chir/o/pod/ist	specialist in hands and feet (now refers just to feet)
8.	Cephal/ic	pertaining to the head
9.	Onych/osis	condition of the nails
10.	Cutane/ous	pertaining to the skin

Section F

1. Formation of eggs

2. Electrical record of the heart

3. Resembling fat

4. Examination of the stomach

5. Measurement of the pelvis

6. Less than normal formation

7. Narrowing of the mitral valve of the heart

8. Destruction of bone

9. Without menstrual flow

10. Formation of blood cells

Section G

1. Bronchiectasia
2. Splenectomy ≠ enlargement → incision
3. Cystography
4. Gynecologist
5. Hemolysis
6. Lithotomy
7. Erythropenia
8. Pathogenic
9. Cardiomegaly
10. Angiotripsy

LESSON 5

Section A

	Meaning	Suffix
1.	Eat	-phagia
2.	Taste	-geusia
3.	Pregnancy	-cyesis
4.	Smell	-osmia
5.	Vision	-opia, -opsy
6.	Touch	-aphia
7.	Breathing	-pnea

Section B

1.	Olfact/ory	pertaining to smell
2.	Opt/ic	pertaining to vision
3.	Audit/ory	pertaining to hearing
4.	Acoust/ic	pertaining to hearing
5.	Bi/o/logy	study of life
6.	Ment/al	pertaining to thinking
7.	Gustat/ory	pertaining to taste
8.	Spir/o/meter	instrument to measure breathing
9.	Men/o/rrhea	menstrual flow
10.	Urin/ary	pertaining to urination

Section C

Element	Example
1. -phoria	euphoria
2. -esthesia	anesthesia
3. -orexia	anorexia
4. -pepsia	dyspepsia
5. -crin-	endocrine
6. -phasia	aphasia
7. Somni-	insomnia
8. Mastico-	masticate
9. Dipso-	dipsomaniac

Section D

1. Movement
2. Touch
3. Breathing
4. Eating
5. Elimination of feces
6. Urination
7. Giving birth
8. Growth
9. Muscle contraction in internal organs

Section E

1. Bad taste
2. Sensation of movement
3. Grow under (another name for pituitary, which grows under the brain)
4. Secrete within (i.e., into the blood)
5. Much thirst
6. Instrument to measure breathing
7. Vision of living tissue
8. More than normal breathing
9. Without speech
10. Woman who has not given birth

Section F

1. Anorexia
2. Euphoria
3. Pseudocyesis
4. Menorrhagia
5. Phagocyte
6. Viviparous
7. Progesterone
8. Auditory
9. Mastication
10. Somnambulism

LESSON 6

Section A

	Prefix	Examples
1.	Hyper-	hypertension
2.	Intra-	intracellular
3.	Micro-	microscope
4.	Ante-	antenatal
5.	Epi-	epidermis
6.	Trans-	transverse
7.	Neo-	neoplasia
8.	Post-	posterior
9.	Eu-	euphonic
10.	Auto-	autoimmune

Section B

1.	Large	macro-
2.	With	syn-
3.	Same	homo-
4.	Half	semi-
5.	Around	circum-
6.	Against	contra-
7.	Below	hypo-

Section C

1. A/pnea   without breathing

2. Dys/pepsia   bad digestion

3. Eu/phoria   good emotional feeling

4. Hyper/esthesia   more than normal physical sensation

5. Endo/crine   secrete within (i.e., into the blood)

6. Dia/physis   grow through

7. An/aphia   without touch

Section D

1. Post/nasal   pertaining to behind the nose

2. Chir/o/pod/ist   specialist in hands and feet (refers now just to feet)

3. Neo/plasia   new (abnormal) formation

4. Spiro/meter   instrument to measure breathing

5. Peri/mast/itis   inflammation around the breast

6. Axill/ary   pertaining to the underarm

7. Dermato/log/ist   specialist in the study of skin

8. Sub/cutane/ous   pertaining to under the skin

9. Pneumo/graph   instrument to record breathing

10. Hypo/derm/ic   pertaining to under the skin

11. Cephal/ic   pertaining to the head

12. Poly/dactyl/y   condition of many digits

13. Auricul/ar   pertaining to the external ear

14. Dys/men/o/rrhea   painful menstrual flow

15. Viscer/al   pertaining to internal organs

Section E

1. Before birth

2. Half paralysis

3. Less than normal formation

4. Across the skin

5. Many breasts

6. Between the ribs

7. Same tone

8. Behind the peritoneum (membrane in abdomen)

9. Through the mouth

10. Against infection

Section F

1. Dysentery

2. Epidermis

3. Intracellular

4. Microscopy

5. Suprarenal

6. Contraception

7. Asthenia

8. Autoimmune

9. Premolar

10. Hyperemia

LESSON 7

Section A

1.	Above	superior
2.	Dividing anterior and posterior	coronal
3.	Back	dorsal
4.	Front	anterior
5.	Below	caudal

Section B

1.	Transverse	6.	Internal
2.	Superficial	7.	Coronal
3.	Proximal	8.	Longitudinal
4.	Sagittal	9.	Distal
5.	Lateral	10.	Medial

Section C

1. Superior, cephalic
2. Inferior, caudal
3. Transverse
4. Lateral
5. Superficial
6. Distal
7. Medial
8. Anterior, ventral
9. Proximal
10. Coronal
11. Posterior, dorsal
12. Inferior, caudal
13. Transverse
14. Lateral
15. Sagittal

LESSON 8

Section A

1. Femoro-
2. Ilio-
3. Cranio-
4. Clavico-
5. Phalango-
6. Costo-
7. Carpo-
8. Rachi-, spino-
9. Sterno-
10. Scapulo-
11. Metacarpo-
12. Humero-
13. Tarso-
14. Tibio-
15. Patello-

Note: From this point on, definitions occasionally will be simplified by omitting "pertaining to" and "condition of."

Section B

1. Poly/myos/itis — inflammation of many muscles
2. Medull/ary — pertaining to marrow
3. Intra/crani/al — within the skull
4. Spondyl/osis — condition of a vertebra
5. Chondro/blast — embryonic cartilage
6. Pelvi/metry — measurement of the pelvis
7. Syn/ovi/al — pertaining to synovium
8. Dis/articul/ar — joints apart
9. Peri/oste/um — something around bone
10. Sub/scapul/ar — under the scapula

11. Coccyg/eal — pertaining to the coccyx

12. Syndesm/osis — bound together (a type of joint)

13. Osteo/lysis — destruction of bone

14. Rachi/an/esthes/ia — lack of sensation in the spine

15. Fasci/ectomy — removal of fascia

16. Peron/eal — pertaining to the fibula

17. Pub/ic sym/physis — pubis; grow with (joint made by pubic bones)

18. Inter/cost/al — between the ribs

19. Myelo/genesis — formation of marrow

20. Arthr/itis — inflammation of joints

21. Osteo/myel/itis — inflammation of bone marrow

22. Sub/stern/al — beneath the sternum

Section C

1. Extracranial
2. Tenosynovitis
3. Syndesmopexy
4. Sarcolemma
5. Perichondrium
6. Costophrenic
7. Carpometacarpal
8. Patelliform
9. Radioulnar
10. Myeloma
11. Myasthenic
12. Rachiodynia
13. Spondylomalacia

LESSON 9

Section A

1. Seizure
2. Herniation
3. Infection
4. Pain
5. Fear
6. Fever
7. Extreme flow
8. Weakness
9. Stone
10. Tumor
11. Fast
12. Stiffness
13. Deficiency
14. Dilatation
15. Stricture

Section B

1. Narco/lepsy   numbness (sleep) seizure
2. An/algesia   without sensation of pain
3. Ankylo/arthr/osis   stiffness of joints
4. Myo/rrhexis   rupture of muscle
5. Patho/genic   producing disease
6. Pyro/phobia   fear of fever (or fire)
7. Hemi/plegia   paralysis of half (of the body)
8. Viscero/ptosis.   sagging of internal organs
9. Osteo/malacia   softening of bones
10. Spondyl/itis   inflammation of a vertebra
11. Cranio/schisis   split skull
12. Anti/sepsis   against infection
13. Myo/spasm   spasm of muscle
14. Meno/rrhagia   extreme menstrual flow
15. Cephalo/megaly   enlargement of head

Section C

1. Displacement of the testis
2. Poison in the blood
3. Kidney stone
4. Narrowing of the esophagus
5. Blood in the urine
6. Pain in the gall bladder
7. Producing disease
8. Nerve weakness
9. Slow reading
10. Characterized by fever

Section D

1. Pyromania
2. Tachycardia
3. Blepharoptosis
4. Arteriosclerosis
5. Myxedema
6. Phleborrhexis
7. Carcinophobia
8. Cystocele
9. Leukopenia
10. Ankyloglossia

LESSON 10

Section A

1.	Kerato/plasty	repair of the cornea (used for corneal transplant)
2.	Cerebr/al mening/itis	inflammation of the meninges of the brain
3.	Neur/asthenia	weakness (inefficiency) of nerves
4.	Encephal/oma	tumor of the brain
5.	Retino/pathy	disease of the retina
6.	Schizo/phren/ia	"split mind" (group of psychoses)
7.	Myelo/gram	record of the spinal cord
8.	Psycho/logy	study of the mind
9.	Myringo/scope	instrument to examine the eardrum
10.	Peri/ophthalm/ic	around the eye
11.	Neur/osis	nervous condition
12.	Intra/ventricul/ar	within the ventricles
13.	Cerebro/spin/al	pertaining to brain and spinal cord
14.	An/encephal/ic	without a (part of the) brain
15.	Conjunctiv/itis	inflammation of the conjunctiva

Section B

1.	Meningosepsis	6.	Medullary
2.	Pontocerebellar	7.	Neurolysis
3.	Otalgia, otodynia	8.	Myelopathy
4.	Meningocele	9.	Neurologist
5.	Lacrimopenia	10.	Myringotomy, tympanotomy

Section C

1.	Pertaining to the pons and medulla	6.	Enzyme in the tears
2.	Around the eye	7.	Specialist in the ear
3.	Alongside the ear	8.	Inflammation of gray matter of the spinal cord
4.	Hardening of the eardrum	9.	Suturing of a nerve
5.	Pertaining to mind and body	10.	Inflammation of the muscles of the eye

Section D

1.	Dacryocystitis	3.	Ventriculography
2.	Retinoscopy	4.	Auriculocranial

5. Otopyorrhea

6. Micrencephaly

7. Cerebrospinal fluid

8. Meningomalacia

9. Neurotherapy

10. Neuratrophia

LESSON 11

1. 1

2. By considering the context in which it is used

3. By considering the context in which it is used

4. Dictionary (from Latin, meaning a saying)

5.

	Meaning	Adjective	Pertaining to
a.	Nerve condition	neurotic	a nerve condition
b.	"Split mind"	schizophrenic	"a split mind"
c.	Instrument to examine small things	microscopic	examining small things
d.	Inflammation of joints	arthritic	inflammation of joints
e.	Measure	metric	measurement
f.	More than normal formation	hyperplastic	more than normal formation
g.	Digits together	syndactylic	fused digits
h.	That which produces cancer	carcinogenic	producing cancer
i.	Destruction of bone	osteolytic	destruction of bone
j.	Skull	cranial	the skull

6.

	Pertaining to	Noun	Meaning
a.	Against infection	antisepsis	against infection
b.	The pubis	pubis	
c.	Formation	genesis	formation
d.	The external ear	auricle	external ear
e.	Without pain	analgesia	without pain
f.	Marrow	medulla	marrow
g.	Bad digestion	dyspepsia	bad digestion
h.	Study of life	biology	study of life
i.	A spasm	spasm	
j.	Numbness	narcosis	numbness

LESSON 12

Section A

1. Hemo/rrhage — extreme flow of blood
2. Spleno/megaly — enlargement of the spleen
3. Cardio/vascul/ar — pertaining to heart and vessels
4. Angio/gram — record of a vessel
5. Coron/ary — pertaining to arteries of heart
6. Phleb/itis — inflammation of a vein
7. Atrio/ventricul/ar — pertaining to atrium and ventricle
8. Arteri/ole — small artery
9. Vaso/dilatation — dilatation of a vessel
10. Hemat/uria — blood in the urine
11. End/o/card/itis — inflammation within the heart
12. Lymph/ang/itis — inflammation of a lymph vessel
13. Sero/logy — study of serum
14. Thymo/lytic — destructive of thymus gland
15. Hemato/poiesis — formation of blood (cells)
16. Spleno/rrhagia — extreme flow (of blood) from spleen
17. Hem/angi/oma — tumor of blood vessel
18. Myo/card/ial — pertaining to heart muscle
19. Ser/ous — pertaining to serum
20. Phleb/ectasia — dilatation of veins

Section B

1. Cardiectasia
2. Interatrial
3. Angioma
4. Arteriosclerosis
5. Sphygmometer (distingush from sphygmomanometer, an instrument to measure blood pressure; mano- = pressure)
6. Splenectomy
7. Cardiopathy

8. Hemolysis

9. Lymphedema

10. Mitrostenosis (usually mitral stenosis)

Section C

1. Without a pulse

2. Tumor of a lymph gland

3. Treatment with serum

4. Hormone that increases pressure in blood vessels

5. Poisonous to the thymus

6. Crushing of a vessel

7. Pain in the spleen

8. Membrane around the heart

9. Blood tumor

10. Disease of capillaries

Section D

1. Cardiorrhexis
2. Plasmapheresis
3. Vasospasm; angiospasm
4. Coronary occlusion
5. Thrombophlebitis
6. Hematocoelia
7. Thymosin
8. Arteriosclerosis
9. Cardiomegaly
10. Hematemesis

REVIEW TEST 1

Section A

"Pertaining to" is understood in all cases.

1. Body cavity
2. External ear
3. Resembling breast
4. Middle of elbow
5. Middle (size) rump
6. Foot
7. Internal organs
8. Skin
9. Sole of foot
10. Cheek
11. Half of spine to head, half of spine to neck
12. Large muscle of breast
13. Upon surface
14. Loin
15. Groin
16. Smell
17. Growing under, secrete within
18. Next to ear

19. Ligament

20. Fibula

21. Between ribs

22. Grow with

23. Marrow

24. Cerebellum, little foot

25. With sides, self-law

26. Atria and ventricles

27. Eardrum

28. Front of brain

29. Around cartilage

30. Joint cavity

31. From a sinew (tendon; the original meaning of neuro-)

32. Hip

33. Near forearm joint

Section B

1.	An/esthe/tic	without sensation
2.	Cephal/odynia	head pain (ache)
3.	Neur/asthenia	nerve weakness (inefficiency)
4.	Hyper/algesia	more than normal sensation of pain
5.	Carcino/genic	producing cancer
6.	Brady/cardia	slow heart (beat)
7.	Phleb/ectasia	dilatation of vein
8.	Coron/ary thromb/osis	clot in artery of heart
9.	Narco/lepsy	numbness (sleep) seizure
10.	Spleno/rrhagia	extreme flow (hemorrhage) from spleen
11.	Angi/oma	tumor of a vessel
12.	Mitr/al stenosis	stricture of mitral valve
13.	Peri/card/itis	inflammation around the heart
14.	Anti/sep/tic	against infection
15.	Arteriol/ar	small artery
16.	My/algia	pain in muscle
17.	Myringo/tomy	incision into eardrum
18.	Ophthalmo/logist	specialist in study of eyes
19.	A/lacrima	without tears
20.	Retino/graphy	record of retina
21.	Hemato/poiesis	formation of blood (cells)
22.	Hemi/an/opia	without vision in half (of eye)
23.	Pelvi/metry	measurement of pelvis

24.	Cardio/vascular	heart and vessels
25.	Dys/kinesia	difficult movement
26.	Intra/cranial	within the skull
27.	Hypo/meno/rrhea	less than normal menstrual flow
28.	In/somnia	without sleep
29.	Cheilo/schisis	split lip
30.	A/phas/ic	without speech
31.	Dipso/mania	obsessive preoccupation (related to) thirst
32.	Osteo/lysis	destruction of bone
33.	Tachy/pnea	fast breathing

Section C

These are the preferred terms.

1. Visceroptosis
2. Vasostenosis
3. Sphygmometer
4. Meningoma
5. Lymphedema
6. Rachimalacia
7. Myorrhexis
8. Hematopenia
9. Pyretic, febrile
10. Anuria
11. Splenogenesis
12. Costosternal
13. Mammogram
14. Omphalocele
15. Hyperdactyly
16. Onychectomy
17. Parietal
18. Hypodermic, subcutaneous
19. Retinopexy
20. Angiotripsy

21. Abiotic
22. Dysodia
23. Femorotibial
24. Pneumograph
25. Exocrine
26. Polyarteritis
27. Megacephalic
28. Postmastectomy
29. Suprascapular
30. Superficial
31. Dorsal
32. Medial
33. Tarsal
34. Distal
35. Sarcophagic
36. Transverse
37. Lithotomy
38. Sagittal
39. Neurotic

LESSON 13

The following are the preferred forms.

1. Meninges
2. Metastases
3. Carpi
4. Angioplasties
5. Axillae
6. Sacra
7. Thoraces
8. Neuroses
9. Costae
10. Hematomas
11. Plexuses
12. Crania
13. Medullae
14. Appendectomies
15. Septa
16. Nares
17. Alveoli
18. Tracheas
19. Nephrons
20. Glottides

LESSON 14

Section A

1. Attachment point
2. Covering
3. Principal part
4. Outer part
5. Small projection
6. Passage
7. Partition
8. Part of organ farthest from exit
9. Branch
10. Network

Section B

1. Psychro/phil/ic — cold-loving
2. Dia/gnosis — through knowledge (identification of disease)
3. Histo/logy — study of tissue
4. Peri/ton/eum — stretch around (serous membrane of abdominal cavity)
5. Aden/oid — resembling a gland
6. Dys/trophy — bad nourishment (producing weakness, wasting)
7. Eu/crasy — good mixture (i.e., health)
8. Chromo/some — color body
9. In/cis/ion — cut in
10. Tubercul/osis — condition with small swellings (a bacterial infection)
11. Cortico/spinal — outer part (of cerebrum) and spinal cord
12. Cryo/genic — producing extreme cold

226

13. Ana/phylaxis   excessive protection (rapid, severe hypersensitive reaction)

14. Myelo/genous   originating in marrow

15. Top/ical   pertaining to place (i.e., local area; refers to skin)

Section C

1. Thermometer

2. Psychrophilic

3. Sarcolemma

4. Atrophy (produces wasting of tissue)

5. Pseudocyesis

6. Adenalgia

7. Chromatography (a technique that separates different kinds of chemical molecules)

8. Cytopenia

9. Somatotrophic (usually somatotropic; stimulates growth)

10. Etiology

Section D

1. Hormone that influences the reproductive organs

2. Enzyme (to digest) fat

3. Middle layer

4. Egg bearer

5. Muscle straight on side of eye

6. Pertaining to destruction of cells

7. Pertaining to same pull

8. Study of nerve tissue

9. Milk sugar

10. Recording of place

Section E

1. Diagnostic

2. Lysosome

3. Seminiferous

4. Hypertrophy

5. Corticosteroids

6. Eupepsia

7. Thermogram

8. Chromophilic

9. Pseudesthetic

10. Prophylaxis

LESSON 15

Section A

1. Stomach
2. Colon (often used for large intestine generally)
3. Liver
4. Rectum and anus
5. Pancreas
6. Tongue
7. Small intestine
8. Esophagus
9. Pharynx
10. Mouth

Section B

1. Palato/schisis — split (cleft) palate
2. Pylor/ic stenosis — stricture of pylorus (sphincter)
3. Duoden/al — pertaining to duodenum
4. Tonsill/ectomy — removal of tonsils
5. Cheilo/rrhaphy — suture of the lip
6. Pharyngo/tympan/ic — pertaining to pharynx and ear
7. Gastro/plegia — paralysis of the stomach (muscles)
8. Dys/enter/y — bad intestine (a variety of inflammatory disorders)
9. Peri/ton/itis — inflammation of peritoneum (which stretches around organs)
10. Chole/litho/tripsy — crushing of a gall (bile) stone
11. Odont/oid — resembling a tooth
12. Stomat/oma — tumor of the mouth
13. Oro/pharynx — (part of) pharynx (adjacent to) mouth
14. Sphincter/algia — pain in a sphincter
15. Ex/odont/ia — removal of a tooth (tooth out)

Section C

1. Glossopharyngeal
2. Proctologist
3. Gastrocele
4. Ileocecal
5. Coloscopy
6. Gingivitis
7. Odontopathy
8. Gastroenteralgia
9. Hepatomegaly
10. Pancreatogenous

Section D

1. Pertaining to teeth and tongue
2. Stone in a tonsil
3. Pertaining to bile in the blood
4. New opening from the appendix

228

5. Through the mouth

6. Stricture of the rectum and anus

7. Pigment of the bile

8. Infection in the intestine

9. Stone in the liver duct

10. Inflammation of the nasopharynx

Section E

1. Cheilophagia

2. Rectopexy

3. Gastrorrhea

4. Cholecystokinin

5. Extraperitoneal

6. Ileocecal

7. Coloptosis

8. Esophagocele

9. Stomatodysodia

10. Hypoglossal

CROSSWORD 1

Digestive System

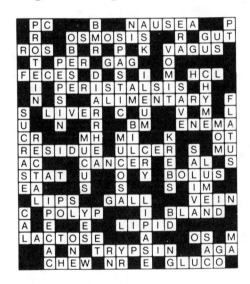

LESSON 16

Section A

1. Colo/stomy — formation of new opening from the colon (large intestine)

2. Thoraco/centesis — puncture of the thorax

3. Spleno/pexy — fixation of the spleen

4. Hemo/stasis — stopping (flow of) blood

5. Psycho/therapy — treatment of the mind

6. Omphalo/tripsy — crushing of the navel (actually the umbilical cord)

7. Kerato/plasty — repair of the cornea

8. Cardio/graphy — recording the heart

9.	Ped/iatric	healing of children
10.	Gastro/clysis	irrigation of the stomach
11.	Pancreato/pexy	fixation of the pancreas
12.	Laparo/tomy	incision into the abdominal wall
13.	Cheilo/rrhaphy	suture of the lip
14.	Hepato/centesis	puncture of the liver
15.	Psych/iatrist	healer of the mind
16.	Ileostomy	formation of new opening from the ileum
17.	Tracheo/tomy	incision into the trachea
18.	Angio/tripsy	crushing of a vessel
19.	Prosth/odontics	addition of teeth
20.	Chole/stasis	stopping (flow of) bile

Section B

1. Splenectomy
2. Pancreatotomy
3. Rhinoplasty
4. Encephalogram
5. Arthroscopy

6. Hydrotherapy
7. Venicentesis (venipuncture also used)
8. Tracheostomy
9. Oroclysis, stomatoclysis
10. Palatorrhaphy

Section C

1. Healing of the feet
2. Pertaining to an addition
3. Irrigation of the colon
4. Fixation of the diaphragm
5. Pertaining to treatment

6. Stopping (flow) of bile
7. Pertaining to stopping (flow) of mucus
8. Removal of a portion of the vas deferens
9. Incision into the kidney
10. Recording of the kidney pelvis

Section D

1. Amniocentesis
2. Homeostasis
3. Cystography
4. Colporrhaphy
5. Otoscopy

6. Thoracotomy
7. Hysterectomy
8. Hemiphalangectomy
9. Ureteroproctostomy
10. Dermatoplasty

LESSON 17

Section A

1. Hypophys/ectomy   removal of the hypophysis
2. Thyro/aden/itis   inflammation of the thyroid gland
3. Epi/glottis   above the glottis
4. Pulmon/ary   pertaining to the lungs
5. Pleuro/scopy   examination of the pleura
6. Phreno/ptosis   sagging of the diaphragm
7. Pancreato/lith   stone in the pancreas
8. Rhino/rrhagia   extreme flow from the nose (nosebleed)
9. Naso/lacrim/al   pertaining to nose and tears
10. Laryngo/plegia   paralysis of the larynx (muscles)
11. Pneumon/ectomy   removal of a lung
12. Phreno/spasm   spasm of the diaphragm
13. Sinus/itis   inflammation of the sinuses
14. Bronchi/ectasia   dilatation of the bronchi
15. Laryngo/cele   herniation of the larynx
16. Alveol/ar   pertaining to the alveoli
17. Adreno/tropic   influencing the adrenal gland
18. Pleur/isy   inflammation of the pleura
19. Tracheo/plasty   repair of the trachea
20. Broncho/pneumon/ia   condition of lungs (beginning in) bronchioles

Section B

1. Thyromegaly (also called goiter)
2. Pancreatoma
3. Oophorocentesis
4. Bronchoscopy
5. Laryngoscope
6. Pleurodynia
7. Pneumonosis
8. Sinogram
9. Pancreatopathy
10. Laryngectomy

Section C

1. External nostrils
2. Condition of pleura and lungs
3. Tumor of the parathyroid
4. Black condition of the lungs
5. Pertaining to around the pharynx
6. Pertaining to within the trachea
7. Disease of the ovary
8. Tumor of the testis
9. Pain in the diaphragm
10. Resembling a sinus

Section D

1. Hypopituitarism
2. Alveolobronchiolitis
3. Adrenocorticotropin
4. Hyperthyroidism
5. Pneumococci
6. Pharyngoxerosis
7. Tracheomalacia
8. Cryptorchidism
9. Phrenicotripsy (phrenico = phrenic nerve)
10. Nasal septum

CROSSWORD 2

Respiration

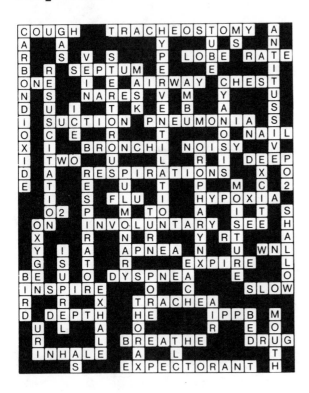

LESSON 18

Section A

1. Oil
2. Saliva
3. Starch
4. Semen
5. Drug
6. Substance
7. Glass
8. Sodium
9. Keratin
10. Potassium

Section B

1. Fat   lipo-
2. Milk   galacto-
3. Salt   sali-
4. Sweat   hidro-
5. Mucus   muco-
6. Pus   puro-
7. Sugar   glyco-
8. Water   hydro-
9. Glue   collo-
10. Air   aero-

Section C

1. Hyal/oid   resembling glass
2. Pneumo/thorax   air in the thorax
3. Lact/ose   milk sugar (carbohydrate)
4. Semini/fer/ous   bearing semen (actually producing sperm)
5. Pyo/genic   producing pus
6. Pharmaco/logy   study of drugs
7. Hyper/hidr/osis   more than normal sweat
8. Glyco/lysis   destruction of glucose
9. Neuro/glia   "nerve glue" (nervous system cells accessory to neurons)
10. Cyto/plasm   substance of cell (other than nucleus)
11. Hypo/kal/emia   less than normal potassium in blood
12. Galactos/emia   galactose in the blood

13. Collagen/ous   producing collagen

14. Sial/o/lith   saliva stone

15. Lipo/lyt/ic   pertaining to break down of fat

Section D

1. Halogen
2. Pyorrhea
3. Polysaccharide
4. Keratocyte
5. Cerolysin
6. Thiourea
7. Sudoriferous
8. Polydipsia
9. Hypernatremia
10. Glycogenesis
11. Hormonopoiesis
12. Enzymuria
13. Fecalith
14. Myxedema
15. Adiposis
16. Seborrheic
17. Mucocolitis
18. Saline
19. Gluconeogenesis
20. Pneumatocardia

LESSON 19

Section A

1. Pyelo/nephr/itis   inflammation of kidney pelvis

2. Uro/cysto/clysis   irrigation of urinary bladder

3. Urethro/stenosis   stricture of urethra

4. Amnio/centesis   puncture of amnion

5. Myo/metr/ium   muscle of uterus

6. Oo/genesis   formation of an egg

7. Orchido/pexy   fixation of testis

8. Phall/ic   pertaining to the penis

9. Perineo/rrhaphy   suture of the perineum

10. Trans/urethr/al   across the urethra

11. Spermato/lysis   destruction of sperm

12. Scroto/cele   herniation of the scrotum

13. Mamill/ary   pertaining to little breast

14. Epi/thel/ium   (tissue) upon the surface

15. Masto/carcin/oma   cancerous tumor of the breast

16. Salpingo/cyesis   tubal pregnancy

17. Gyneco/mastia   breast like a woman

18. Uretero/lith   stone in the ureter

19. Supra/ren/al   above the kidney

20. Hystero/salpingo/   removal of the uterus, tubes, and ovaries
    oophor/ectomy

Section B

1. Gonorrhea (a bacterial infection)
2. Mastoid
3. Epididymitis
4. Vasectomy
5. Cystography

6. Salpingo-oophoritis
7. Gynecologist
8. Ureterotomy
9. Cystalgia
10. Colpectasia

Section C

1. Many men (husbands)
2. Pertaining to bladder and perineum
3. Incision into the prepuce
4. Producing female characteristics
5. Tumor of the penis
6. Enlargement of the prostate
7. Recording of the uterine tube
8. Abnormal condition of tissue usually inside uterus
9. Rupture of the amnion
10. Gland located above the kidney

Section D

1. Gonad
2. Polythelia
3. Episioplasty
4. Vulvovaginitis
5. Perineocele

6. Urethratresia
7. Amastia
8. Ookinesia
9. Placentoma
10. Pyeloplication

LESSON 20

Section A

1. Pit
2. Isolated part
3. Arch
4. Crossing point
5. Internal fold
6. Depressed area
7. Opening
8. Thin layer
9. Small sac
10. Cavity of hollow organ

Section B

1. Tox/emia — poison in the blood
2. Idio/path/ic — "one's own" disease (used when cause is unknown)
3. Dermato/myc/osis — fungous condition of skin
4. Ger/iatr/ic — healing of (problems related to) old age
5. Ankylo/dactyl/ia — stiffening of digits
6. Bacteri/cid/al — killing bacteria
7. My/asthenia — weakness of muscle
8. Xer/ophthalm/ia — dry eyes
9. Pro/gnosis — know before (i.e., predict)
10. Chor/oid — resembling membrane
11. Radiculo/tomy — cutting the root (of a spinal nerve)
12. Crypt/orchid/ism — hidden testis (undescended)
13. Circum/cis/ion — cutting around (to remove prepuce)
14. Strati/fied — layered
15. Striat/ed — striped
16. Spermi/cid/al — pertaining to killing sperm
17. Chole/ster/ol — solid bile
18. Necr/otic — pertaining to dead condition
19. Hyper/bar/ic — pertaining to more than normal pressure
20. Mening/o/cocci — spherical (bacteria infecting) the meninges

Section C

1. Necrophobia
2. Staphylococcus
3. Atrichous

4. Barometer

5. Ataxia (lack of muscle coordination)

6. Neurasthenia (weakness due to inefficient nerves)

7. Ergogram (made during muscular exertion)

8. Transluminal

9. Peri-insular

10. Mycotoxin

11. Acromegaly

12. Gerontology

13. Infundibuloma

14. Intervertebral foramen

15. Mycostatic

16. Pedodontist

LESSON 21

Section A

1. Blue
2. Gray
3. Black
4. Yellow
5. White
6. Greenish-gray
7. Yellow-orange
8. Yellow
9. Purple
10. Red

Section B

1. Thick
2. Straight
3. Large
4. Wide
5. Smooth
6. Rough
7. Short
8. Straight
9. Small
10. Twisted

Section C

1. Brachy/dactyl/y   short digits
2. Micr/ophthalm/ia   small eyes
3. Melan/oma   black tumor
4. Corpus luteum   yellow body

5. Macro/phage   big eater (type of phagocyte)

6. Dolicho/cephal/ic   long head (anterior to posterior)

7. Leuko/cyt/osis   condition of white cells (temporary increase in number)

8. Cyan/osis   blue condition

9. Orth/odont/ist   specialist in straightening teeth

10. Platy/rrhine   broad-nosed

11. Rectus abdominis   straight (on the) abdomen

12. Polio/myel/itis   inflammation of gray (matter of the) spinal cord

13. Scolio/rach/itis   twisted vertebral column (-itis was formerly used for condition)

14. Eury/opia   wide (space between) the eyes

15. Leio/derm/ia   smooth skin

16. Erythro/cyto/poiesis   formation of red cells

Section D

1. Leiomyoma
2. Leukodermic
3. Leptomeningoma
4. Polioencephalopathy
5. Glaucoma
6. Erythropenia
7. Macrodontia
8. Melanemesis
9. Cyanopsia
10. Brachycheilia
11. Oxyphilic
12. Streptococcal
13. Trachoma
14. Orthopedic
15. Pachyonychia
16. Micromastia
17. Eurycephalic
18. Xanthochromia
19. Platypodia
20. Stenostomia
21. Megalocheiria

LESSON 22

Section A

1. double
2. ten
3. hundred
4. many much
5. all
6. one
7. more
8. half
9. triple
10. four

Section B

1. milli-
2. mio-, meio-, hypo-
3. hemi-, semi-
4. haplo-
5. tri-
6. nulli-
7. oligo-
8. di-, bi-
9. centi-, hecto-
10. pan-, pant-

Section C

1. mei/osis — condition of a lesser number (of chromosomes)
2. triplo/blast/ic — triple (-layered) embryo
3. hemi/pleg/ia — paralysis of half (of the body)
4. nulli/par/ous — giving birth to none
5. pan/cyto/penia — deficiency of all (blood) cells
6. hypo/therm/ia — less heat (lower body temperature)
7. mono/nucle/osis — condition of (cells with) one nucleus (abnormal increase in number of monocytes)
8. Deci/meter — one-tenth of a meter
9. Dipl/opia — double vision
10. Tri/orchid/ism — three testes
11. Panto/phobia — fear of all (everything)
12. Uni/later/al — one-sided
13. Olig/odont/ia — few teeth
14. Hyper/glycos/uria — extremely large amounts of glucose in urine

Section D

1. Polycythemia
2. Hemipneumonectomy
3. Pleochromatism
4. Oliguria
5. Pancytopenia
6. Multiarticular
7. Monomyoplegia
8. Unisexual
9. Tricuspid
10. Hectoliter
11. Binaural
12. Dichromatopsia
13. Haploid
14. Oligomenorrhea
15. Quadrilateral
16. Tetrasaccharide
17. Hypocholesterolemia
18. Hyperbilirubinemia
19. Centiliter
20. Panosteitis

REVIEW TEST 2

Section A

Words in parentheses explain elements you have not studied or elements that are understood.

1. Cavernous (spongy) bodies

2. Point where (structures) attach to lung

3. Network (of nerves) pertaining to arm

4. Covering of skeletal muscle (fiber)

5. Larger enlargement on humerus

6. Outer passage of ear

7. Part of stomach farthest from exit

8. (Clear) partition

9. Branch of the ischium

10. Stretcher of the muscle covering on the side (of the thigh)

11. Under the tongue (surface); serves tongue muscles

12. (From) pharynx (to) ear

13. Inner nostrils

14. Next to the thyroid

15. Valve at the pylorus (of the stomach)

16. Small projection in the kidney

17. Sperm-bearing

18. Over the glottis

19. Pleura (associated with) organ; in this case, the lung

20. (Supplying) the diaphragm

21. Gland growing under (the brain)

22. "Nerve glue" (tissue in nervous system)

23. Sweat-bearing

24. Glassy (in that it is transparent)

25. Cell substance (other than nucleus)

26. Oily

27. Muscle of uterus

28. Small breast-like (structures of brain)

29. Resembling membrane

30. Fat around kidney

31. Depression in the front of the skull

32. Lobe isolated (from the surface) of the brain

33. Cavity of a vein

34. Folds inside the bladder

35. Striped (appearance of fibers)

36. Moving hairs (to produce gooseflesh)

37. First branch to the back

38. Small network

39. Pertaining to tongue

40. Middle of intestine (connecting it to body wall)

41. Horny layer (literal meaning of corn-)

42. Crossing-over point of nerves for vision

43. Thin layers

44. Around muscle

45. Part of pharynx (adjoining) nose

46. Full of collagen (a protein that produces glue)

47. Glassy

48. Small bladder for semen

49. Broad, flat

50. Belly-leg (from shape)

51. Half tendinous

52. Middle layer

Section B

1. Throw beyond (implies change)

2. Enzyme (to digest) starch

3. Sweet carbohydrate (sugar)

4. Destructive body (has digestive enzymes)

5. Stopping (flow of) blood

6. Pertaining to small air sacs

7. Influencing the adrenal cortex, outer part (of gland located) toward the kidney

8. Many sugars

9. Salt (solution) having the same strength (another use of -ton-)

10. Enlargement of extremities

11. Producing milk

12. Condition of less (in this case, chromosomes)

13. Yellow body

14. Formation of reproductive cells

15. Above the kidney

16. Mucous swelling

17. Influencing the reproductive organs

18. Condition of cell eating

19. Destruction of blood

20. In favor of pregnancy (another use of pro-)

21. Small nuclei

Section C

1.	Dys/crasia	"bad mixture" (used for blood disorders)
2.	Dia/gnost/ic	through knowledge
3.	All/erg/y	"other work" (foreign substances cause reaction)
4.	Hyper/trophy	more than normal nutrition (therefore, increase in size of cells)
5.	Gastro/clysis	irrigation of the stomach
6.	Laparo/rrhaphy	suture of abdominal wall
7.	Pod/iatrist	healer of feet
8.	My/om/ectomy	removal of muscle tumor
9.	Bili/ary stasis	stopping (flow of) bile
10.	Hidr/aden/itis	inflammation of sweat gland
11.	Olig/uria	little (amount of) urine
12.	Saccharo/myces	sugar fungus
13.	Muco/col/itis	mucous inflammation of the colon
14.	Pharmaco/peia	production of drugs
15.	Sialo/phagia	swallowing saliva
16.	Trans/urethr/al prostat/ectomy	removal of prostate through the urethra
17.	Hyster/odynia	pain in the uterus
18.	Bary/phon/ia	heavy (thick) sound (voice)
19.	Cyan/otic	bluish
20.	Megalo/mania	excessive preoccupation (with one's largeness, supposed greatness)

21. Hepato/cirrhosis   yellow-orange condition of liver

22. An/osmia   without smell

23. Strepto/cocc/al   pertaining to spherical cells (in a) twisted (chain)

24. Panto/phobia   fear of everything

25. Pleo/cyt/osis   condition of more cells

26. Electro/phor/esis   carry by electricity (to separate molecules)

27. Cac/odontia   bad teeth

26. Pro/phylaxis   protect before (i.e., prevention of disease)

29. Phalango/tripsy   crushing of a phalanx

30. Bronchiol/itis   inflammation of a small bronchus

Section D

These are the preferred terms.

1. Chromatography

2. Etiology

3. Pseudocyesis

4. Cholecystitis

5. Pyorrhea

6. Esophagocele

7. Amniocentesis

8. Hemipneumectomy

9. Phrenospasm

10. Hyperpituitarism

11. Chondromalacia

12. Hyponatremia

13. Choleliths (cholelithiasis, if thinking of a condition)

14. Polymyalgia

15. Colposcope

16. Pneumomycoses

17. Toxemia

18. Xeroderma

19. Glaucoma

20. Platyonychia

21. Leiomyoma

22. Dichromatism

23. Schizophrenia

24. Pediatric

Glossary-Index
of Word Elements

(G) = Greek origin   (ME) = Middle English origin

(L) = Latin origin   (F) = French origin

Word Element	Meaning	Page
(G) a-	without	31
(L) abdomino-	abdomen	10
(G) -ac	pertaining to	19
(G) acoustico-	hearing	25
(G) acro-	extremity	159
(L) ad-	toward	31
(G) adeno-	gland	101
(L) adipo-	fat	138
(L) adreno-	adrenal (suprarenal)	127
(G) aero-	air	137
(L) -al	pertaining to	19
(G) -algesia	sensation of pain	57
(G) -algia	pain	57
(G) allo-	other	101
(L) alveol-	alveolus	127
(L) ambi-	both	101
(L) amnio-	amnion	45
(G) amylo-	starch	137
(G) an-	without	31
(G) ana-	up	31
(G) andro-	man	145
(G) angio-	vessel	83
(G) ankylo-	stiffness, adhesion	57, 159
(L) ano-	anus	111
(L) ante-	before	31
(L) antebrachium	forearm	111

245

Word Element	Meaning	Page
(G) anterior	front	37
(G) anti-	against	31
(G) -aphia	touch	26
(G) apo-	from	31
(L) appendico-	appendix	111
(L) aqueo-	water	138
(L) -ar	pertaining to	19
(L) arterio-	artery	83
(G) arthro-	joint	45
(L) articulo-	joint	45
(L) -ary	pertaining to	19
(G) -ase	enzyme	19, 101
(G) -asthenia	weakness	57
(L) atrio-	atrium	83
(L) audito-	hearing	25
(L) auriculo-	external ear	9, 69
(L) auriculo-	auricular appendage of atrial wall	83
(G) auto-	self	31
(G) autonomo-	autonomic	69
(L) axilla	underarm	11
(G) baro-	pressure	159
(G) bary-	heavy	166
(G) bi-	two	171
(L) bili-	bile	109
(G) bio-	living	25
(G) -blast	embryonic	101
(G) bol-	throw	159
(L) brachio-	arm	11
(G) brachy-	short	166
(G) brady-	slow	57
(G) broncho-, bronchi-	bronchus	127
(L) bucco-	cheek	9
(G) caco-	bad	101
(L) calculo-	stone	58

Word Element	Meaning	Page
(L) capillaro-	capillary	83
(L) capito-	head	9
(G) carcino-	cancer	57
(G) cardio-	heart	83
(L) carpo-	wrist	11, 48
(G) cata-	down	31
(L) caudal	below	39
(L) ceco-	cecum	111
(G) -cele	herniation	57
(G) celo-	celom	12
(G) -centesis	puncture	121
(L) centi-	one-hundredth	171
(G) cephalic	above	39
(G) cephalo-	head	9
(L) cer-	oil, wax	138
(L) cerebello-	cerebellum	69
(L) cerebro-	cerebrum	69
(L) cervico-	neck	9
(G) cheilo-	lip	9, 107
(G) cheiro-	hand	11
(G) chiasma	crossing point	159
(G) chiro-	hand	11
(G) chole-	bile, gall	109
(G) chondro-	cartilage	45
(G) chorio-	membrane	159
(G) chromo-, chromato-	color	101
(L) -cid-	kill	159
(L) circum-	around	32, 159
(G) cirrho-	yellow-orange	165
(L) -cis-	cut	101
(G) -clast	break down	19
(L) clavico-	clavicle	47
(G) cleido-	clavicle	47
(G) -clysis	irrigation	121
(G) -cnemo-	leg	12

Word Element	Meaning	Page
(G) cocco-	spherical cell	159
(G) coccygo-	coccyx	47
(G) cochleo-	cochlea	71
(G) coelo-	coelom	12
(G) colla-	glue	137
(L) collo-	neck	9
(G) colo-	colon	111
(G) colpo-	vagina	145
(L) con-	with, together	32
(L) conjunctivo-	conjunctiva	71
(L) contra-	against	31
(L) corneo-	cornea	71
(L) coronal	dividing anterior and posterior	39
(L) corono-	arteries of heart	83
(L) corpus	principal part	101
(L) cortico-	cortex	101
(L) costo-	rib	48
(L) coxo-	hip	12
(G) cranio-	cranium	47
(G) -cras-	mixture	101
(G) -crin-	secretion	26
(L) crur-	leg	12
(G) cryo-	cold	103
(G) crypto-	hidden	159
(L) cubito-	elbow	11
(L) cutaneo-	skin	12
(G) cyano-	blue	165
(G) -cyesis	pregnancy	26
(G) cysto-	bladder	109, 143
(G) cyto-	cell	102
(G) dacryo-	tears	71
(G) dactylo-	digit	11
(G) deca-	ten	171
(L) deci-	one-tenth	171
(ME) deep	away from surface	39

Word Element	Meaning	Page
(L) defeca-	elimination of feces	26
(L) dento-	teeth	107
(G) dermo-, dermato-	skin	12
(L) dextral	right	39
(G) di-	two	171
(G) dia-	through	31
(G) diplo-	double	171
(G) -dipsia	thirst	26
(G) dipso-	thirst	26
(L) dis-	apart	31
(L) distal	far from	37
(G) dolicho-	long	166
(L) dormi-	sleeping	25
(L) dorsal	back	37
(L) duodeno-	duodenum	109
(G) dys-	bad, difficult, painful	31
(L) -eal	pertaining to	19
(G) -ectasia, -ectasis	dilatation	19, 57
(G) ecto-	outside	31
(G) -ectomy	excision, removal	19, 121
(G) -ectopia, -ectopy	displacement	57
(G) edema	swelling	57
(G) -emia	condition of blood	58
(G) en-	in	31
(G) encephalo-	brain	69
(G) endo-	inside	31
(G) entero-	intestine	109
(G) ento-	inside	31
(G) enzymo-	enzyme	137
(G) epi-	upon	31
(G) epididymo-	epididymis	149
(G) episio-	area of female external openings	145
(G) -erg-	work	159
(G) erythro-	red	165

Word Element	Meaning	Page
(G) esophago-	esophagus	109
(G) -esthesia	physical sensation	25
(G) eti-	cause	102
(G) eu-	good, normal, healthy	31, 102
(G) eury-	wide	166
(G) ex-, exo-	out, away	32
(G) external	outside	39
(L) extra-	more than, outside of	32
(L) extrinsic	on outside of structure in body	39
(L) fascio-	fascia	47
(L) febri-	fever	59
(L) fecalo-	feces	137
(L) femoro-	thigh	12
(L) femoro-	femur	48
(L) -fer-	carry, bear	102
(L) fibulo-	fibula	48
(L) follicle	small sac or cavity	159
(L) foramen	opening	159
(L) fornix	arch	160
(L) fossa	depressed area	160
(L) fovea	pit	160
(L) frontal	dividing anterior and posterior	39
(L) fundus	part of organ farthest from exit	102
(G) galacto-	milk	137
(G) gamo-	gamete	149
(G) ganglio-	ganglion	69
(G) gastro-	stomach	109
(G) -genesis	production, formation	19
(G) -genic	producing, forming	19
(G) -genous	place of origin	102
(L) genu-	knee	12
(G) geri-, geronto-	old age	160
(L) gest-	pregnancy	26
(G) -geusia	taste	26

Word Element	Meaning	Page
(L) gingivo-	gums	107
(G) glauco-	greenish-gray, silvery	165
(G) -glia	glue	137
(G) glosso-	tongue	107
(G) glott-	glottis	125
(G) gluco-	sugar	137
(G) gluteo-	rump	12
(G) glyco-	sugar	137
(G) -gnosis	knowledge	102, 160
(G) gono-	gonad	149
(G) -gram	record	20
(G) -graph	instrument to record	19
(G) -graphy	recording	19, 121
(L) gusto-	taste	26
(G) gyneco-	woman	145
(G) halo-	salt	137
(G) haplo-	single	171
(G) hecto-	hundred	171
(G) hemi-	half	32, 172
(G) hemo-, hemato-, hema-	blood	83
(G) hepato-	liver	109
(G) hetero-	different, other	32
(G) hidro-	sweat	137
(L) hilum, hilus	attachment point	102
(G) histo-, histi-	tissue	102
(G) homeo-	similar	32
(G) homo-	same	32
(G) hormono-	hormone	138
(L) humero-	humerus	48
(G) hyalo-	glass	138
(G) hydro-	water	138
(G) hyper-	more than normal	32, 172
(G) hypo-	under, less than normal	32, 172
(G) hypophyseo-	hypophysis (pituitary)	127
(G) hystero-	uterus	145

Word Element	Meaning	Page
(G) -ia	condition, process	20
(G) -iasis	condition (often abnormal)	20
(G) -iatrist	healer	121
(G) -iatry	healing	121
(G) -ic	pertaining to	19
(G) idio-	one's own	160
(L) ileo-	ileum	109
(L) ilio-	ilium	49
(L) in-	into, not	32
(L) inferior	below	39
(L) infra-	below	32
(L) infundibulum	funnel-shaped tube	160
(L) inguino-	inguinal area	11
(L) insula	isolated	160
(L) integumento-	skin	12
(L) inter-	between	32
(L) internal	inside	39
(L) intra-	within	32
(L) intrinsic	belonging entirely to one structure	39
(G) ischio-	ischium	49
(G) -ism	condition (often abnormal)	20
(G) iso-	same	32
(G) -ist	specialist	20
(G) -itis	inflammation	20, 58
(L) jejuno-	jejunum	109
(L) kal-	potassium	138
(G) kerato-	cornea	71
(G) kerato-	keratin	138
(G) kilo-	thousand	171
(G) -kinesia	movement	25
(L) labio-	lip	9, 107
(L) lacrimo-	tears	71
(L) lacto-	milk	137
(L) lamella	thin layer	160

Word Element	Meaning	Page
(L) lamina	layer	160
(G) laparo-	abdominal wall	11
(G) laryngo-	larynx	125
(L) lateral	side	37
(G) leio-	smooth	166
(G) -lemma	covering	102
(G) -lepsy	seizure	58
(G) lepto-	thin	166
(G) leuco-, leuko-	white	165
(L) linguo-	tongue	107
(G) lipo-	fat	138
(G) -lith	stone	58
(G) litho-	stone	58
(G) -logist	specialist in the study	20
(G) -logy	study	20
(L) longitudinal	lengthwise	39
(L) lumbo-	lumbar area	11
(L) lumen	cavity of hollow organ	160
(L) luteo-	yellow	165
(L) lympho-	lymph	83
(G) -lysis	decomposition, destruction	20, 58
(G) macro-	large	32, 166
(L) mal-	bad	32, 101
(G) -malacia	softening	58
(L) mamilli-	nipple	145
(L) mammo-	breast	11, 145
(G) mania	obsessive preoccupation	58
(L) manu-	hand	11
(L) mastico-	chewing	26
(G) masto-	breast	11, 145
(L) meatus	passage	102
(L) medial	middle	37
(L) medullo-	marrow	47
(L) medullo-	medulla	69

Word Element	Meaning	Page
(G) megalo-	large	32, 166
(G) -megaly	enlargement	20, 58
(G) meio-	less	172
(G) melano-	black	165
(G) meningo-	meninges	69
(G) meno-	menstruation	26
(L) mento-	thinking, mind	25, 69
(L) mento-	chin	9
(L) mesial	middle	37
(G) meta-	beyond (in degree or position)	32
(G) metacarpo-	metacarpus	48
(G) metatarso-	metatarsus	48
(G) -meter	instrument to measure	20
(G) metro-	uterus	145
(G) -metry	measurement	20
(G) micro-	small	32, 166
(L) milli-	one-thousandth	171
(G) mio-	less	172
(L) mitro-	mitral valve	83
(G) mono-	one	171
(L) morb-	disease	58
(L) mort-	death	160
(L) muco-	mucus	138
(L) multi-	many, much	172
(G) myco-	fungus	160
(G) myelo-	marrow	47
(G) myelo-	spinal cord	69
(G) myo-	muscle	47
(L) myringo-	eardrum	69
(G) myxo-	mucus	138
(G) narco-	numbness	58
(L) naris	nostril	125
(L) naso-	nose	9, 125
(L) natr-	sodium	138

Word Element	Meaning	Page
(G) necro-	death	160
(G) neo-	new	32
(G) nephro-	kidney	143
(G) neuro-, neuri-	nerve	69
(L) nucleo-	central structure	160
(L) nulli-	none	172
(L) oculo-	eye	9, 71
(G) odonto-	teeth	107
(G) -odynia	pain	57
(G) -oid	resembling	20
(G) olecrano-	elbow	11
(L) olfacto-	smell	25
(G) oligo-	few, little	172
(G) -oma	tumor	58
(G) omphalo-	umbilicus	11
(G) onco-	tumor	58
(G) onycho-	nail	12
(G) oo-	egg	145
(G) oophoro-	ovary	127, 145
(G) ophthalmo-	eye	9, 71
(G) -opia, -opsy	vision	25
(G) opto-, optico-	vision	25
(G) orchido-	testis	127, 145
(G) orchio-	testis	145
(G) -orexia	appetite	26
(L) oro-	mouth	107
(G) ortho-	straight	166
(L) -ory	pertaining to	19
(L) -ose	full of	20, 102
(F) -ose	carbohydrate	102
(G) -osis	condition (often abnormal)	20, 58
(G) -osmia	smell	25
(G) osteo-	bone	45
(G) -ostomy	formation of new opening	122

Word Element	Meaning	Page
(G) oto-	ear	69
(L) -ous	pertaining to	19
(L) -ous	full of	20
(L) ovario-	ovary	127, 145
(L) ovo-	egg	145
(G) oxy-	sharp, acid, fast	166
(G) pachy-	thick	166
(L) palato-	palate	107
(G) pan-, pant-	all	172
(G) pancreato-	pancreas	109, 127
(L) papilla	small projection	102
(G) para-	beside, beyond, abnormal	32
(G) parathyro-	parathyroid	127
(L) parieto-	wall of body cavity	12
(L) par-	giving birth	26
(L) patello-	patella	48
(G) patho-	disease	58
(G) -pathy	disease	58
(L) pectoro-	chest	11
(L) pedo-	foot	12
(G) pedo-	child	160
(L) pelvi-, pelvo-	pelvis	49
(G) -penia	deficiency	20, 58
(G) -pepsia	digestion	26
(L) per-	through	31
(G) peri-	around	32
(G) perineo-	perineum	149
(G) peristalsis	muscle contraction in internal organs	26
(G) peritoneo-	peritoneum	109
(G) peroneo-	fibula	48
(G) -pexy	fixation	121
(G) -phagia	eating, swallowing	26
(G) phago-	eating, swallowing	26
(G) phalango-	phalanges	48

Word Element	Meaning	Page
(G) phallo-	penis	149
(G) pharmaco-	drug	138
(G) pharyngo-	pharynx	107, 125
(G) -phasia	speech	25
(G) -philia	affinity, love	102
(G) phlebo-	vein	83
(G) -phobia	fear	58
(G) -phon-	sound	160
(G) -phor-	carry, bear	102
(G) -phoria	emotional feeling	25
(G) phreno-	diaphragm	127
(G) phreno-	mind	69
(G) -phylaxis	protection	102
(G) -physis	growth	26
(L) pilo-	hair	161
(L) pituit-	pituitary (hypophysis)	127
(L) placento-	placenta	145
(L) plantar	sole of foot	12
(G) -plasia	formation (often abnormal)	20
(G) -plasm	substance	138
(G) plasmo-	plasma	84
(G) -plasty	repair, plastic surgery	20, 121
(G) platy-	flat, broad	166
(G) -plegia	paralysis	59
(G) pleo-	more	172
(G) pleuro-	pleura	127
(G) plexus	network	102
(G) -pnea	breathing	26
(G) pneuma-, pneumato-	air	137
(G) pneumo-, pneumono-	lung	127
(G) podo-	foot	12
(G) -poiesis	formation (usually on a continuing basis)	20
(G) polio-	gray	165
(G) poly-	many, much	32, 172
(L) ponto-	pons	69

Word Element	Meaning	Page
(L) popliteal	back of knee	12
(L) post-	behind, after	32
(L) posterior	back	37
(L) pre-	in front of, before	32
(L) preputio-	prepuce	149
(G) pro-	in front of, before	32
(G) procto-	rectum and anus	111
(G) prostato-	prostate gland	149
(G) prostho-	addition	121
(L) proximal	near to	37
(G) pseudo-	false	103
(G) psycho-	mind	69
(G) psychro-	cold	103
(G) -ptosis	drooping	59
(G) ptyalo-	saliva	138
(L) pubo-	pubis	49
(L) pulmo-, pulmono-	lung	127
(L) puro-	pus	138
(L) purpuri-	purple	165
(G) pyelo-	kidney pelvis	143
(G) pyloro-	pylorus	109
(G) pyo-	pus	138
(G) pyro-, pyreto-	fever	59
(L) quadri-	four	171
(G) rachi-, rachio-	spinal column, vertebral column	47
(L) radiculo-	root	160
(L) radio-	radius	48
(L) ramus	branch	103
(L) recto-	straight	103, 166
(L) recto-	rectum	111
(L) reno-	kidney	143
(L) reti-	network	103
(L) retino-	retina	71
(L) retro-	behind, after	32

Word Element	Meaning	Page
(G) rhino-	nose	9, 125
(G) -rrhagia	extreme flow	59
(G) -rrhaphy	suture	121
(G) -rrhea	flow	20
(G) -rrhexis	rupture	59
(L) ruga	fold	160
(G) saccharo-	sugar	137
(L) sacro-	sacrum	47
(L) sagittal	dividing right and left	39
(L) sali-	salt	137
(G) salpingo-	uterine (fallopian) tube	145
(G) sarco-	skeletal muscle	47
(L) scapulo-	scapula	47
(G) -schisis	splitting	59
(G) schizo-	splitting	59
(G) -sclerosis	hardening	59
(G) scolio-	twisted	166
(G) -scope	instrument to examine	20
(G) -scopy	examination	20, 121
(L) scroto-	scrotum	149
(L) sebo-	oil, wax	138
(L) semi-	half, partly	32, 172
(L) semino-	semen	138, 149
(G) -sepsis	infection	59
(L) septum	partition	103
(L) sero-	serum	84
(G) sialo-	saliva	138
(L) sinistral	left	39
(L) sino-, sinus	sinus	125
(G) somato-	body	103
(G) -some	body	103
(L) somni-	sleeping	25
(G) -spasm	spasm	59
(G) spermato-	sperm	149

Word Element	Meaning	Page
(G) sphincter	valve	109
(G) sphyx-, sphygmo-	pulse	83
(L) spino-	spinal column, vertebral column	47
(L) spino-	spinal cord	69
(L) spiro-	breathing	26
(G) splanchno-	viscera	12
(G) spleno-	spleen	83
(G) spondylo-	vertebra	47
(G) staphylo-	cluster	161
(G) -stasis	stopping, standing still	122
(G) steno-	narrow	166
(G) -stenosis	constriction, narrowing, stricture	20, 59
(G) stereo-	solid	161
(G) sterno-	sternum	48
(G) stetho-	chest	11
(G) -sthenia	strength	161
(G) stomato-	mouth	107
(G) -stomy	formation of new opening	21, 122
(L) stratum	layer	161
(G) strepto-	twisted	166
(L) stria	stripe	161
(L) sub-	below	32
(L) sudori-	sweat	137
(L) super-	above, more than	32
(L) superficial	toward the surface	39
(L) superior	above	39
(L) supra-	above, more than	32
(L) suprareno-	suprarenal (adrenal) gland	127
(G) syn-	with, together	32
(G) syndesmo-	ligament	47
(G) synovio-	joint fluid	47
(G) tachy-	fast	59
(L) tacto-	touch	26
(G) tarso-	tarsus	12, 48

Word Element	Meaning	Page
(G) taxo-	order	161
(L) teno-, tendino-	tendon	47
(L) tens-	stretch, pull	103
(L) testi-	testis	127, 145
(G) tetra-	four	171
(G) thelo-	nipple	11, 145
(G) -therapy	treatment	122
(G) thermo-	heat	103
(G) thio-	sulfur	138
(G) thoraco-	thorax	9
(G) thymo-	thymus gland	83
(G) thyro-	thyroid gland	127
(L) tibio-	tibia	48
(G) -tomy	incision	21, 122
(L) -ton-	stretch, pull	103
(L) tonsillo-	tonsil	109
(G) -top-	place	103
(G) toxico-	poison	161
(G) tracheo-	trachea	127
(G) trach-, trachy-	rough	166
(L) trans-	across, through	32
(L) transverse	dividing superior and inferior	39
(G) tri-	three	171
(G) tricho-	hair	161
(G) triplo-	triple	171
(G) -tripsy	crushing, friction	21, 122
(G) -trop-	turn, influence	103
(G) -troph	nourish	103
(L) tuber	swelling, enlargement	103
(L) tunic	covering	102
(G) tympano-	eardrum	69
(L) ulno-	ulna	48
(L) umbilico-	umbilicus	11
(L) uni-	one	171

Word Element	Meaning	Page
(G) uretero-	ureter	143
(G) urethro-	urethra	143
(G) -uria	condition of urine	59
(G) urino-	urination	26
(L) utero-	uterus	145
(L) vagino-	vagina	145
(L) vaso-	vessel	83
(L) vaso-	vas deferens	149
(L) veno-	vein	83
(L) ventral	front	37
(L) ventriculo-	ventricle	69, 83
(L) vesico-	bladder	143
(L) viscero-	viscera	12
(L) vitreo-	glass	138
(L) vulva	area of female external openings	145
(G) xantho-	yellow	165
(G) xero-	dry	161
(G) -y	condition, process	20

INDEX

Italicized numbers indicate illustrations.
Variant spellings and plurals are given
in parentheses.

Duodenal, 112
Duodenal ulcer, 109
Duodenitis, 176
Duodenum, *110*
Dyscrasia, 188
Dysentery, 31, 109, 112
Dysgeusia, 29
Dyskinesia, 95
Dysmenorrhea, 3, 34
Dyspepsia, 26, 34
Dyspeptic, 79
Dysphagia, 176
Dyspnea, 176
Dystrophy, 105

Ectopic 57
Ectoplasm, 31
Edema, 158, 176
Edematous, 57
Efferent arteriole, *144*
Ejaculatory duct, 143
Electric, 19
Electrocardiogram, 3, 24, 83
Electrocardiographic, 92
Electrophoresis, 188
Elixir, 178
Embolism, 176
Embolus(i), 158, 159
Emetic, 179
Encephalitis, 69
Encephaloma, 72
Endarterectomy, 119
Endocarditis, 85, 98
Endocrine, 26, 29, 31, 34, 67, 125
Endocrinology, 176
Endogenous, 92, 102, 182
Endometriosis, 151, 176
Endometrium, 78, 143, *146*, *147*
Endorphin, 182
Endoscopic, 136
Endoscopy, 136
Endosteal, 65
Endotracheal, 130
Energy, 159
Entangle, 31
Enteritis, 176
Enterosepsis, 113
Enzymes, 81
Epidermis, 31, 186
Epididymis(ides), 97, 143, *148*
Epigastric, 92, 158
Epiglottis, *126*, 129, 186
Epilepsy, 58
Epinephrine, 91, 187
Epinephros, 151
Epithelium, 93, 150
Erythrocytes, 81, 165
Erythrocytopoiesis, 168
Esophageal, 136
Esophagitis, 176
Esophagostenosis, 61
Esophagus, 107, *108*, *126*
Etiology, 102, 176
Etymology, 1

Eucrasy, 105
Euphonious, 102
Euphoria, 25, 31, 34
Euryopia, 168
Eustachian tube, *70*
Euthanasia, 102
Excision, 101
Exenteration, 136
Exodontia, 112
Exogenous, 92
Exotic, 32
Expectorate, 11
External abdominal oblique muscle,
    54, 55
External acoustic (auditory) meatus,
    70, 185
External os, *146*
Extensor carpi radialis muscles, *54, 55*
Extensor carpi ulnaris muscle, *55*
Extensor digitorum muscles, *54, 55*
Extrasensory, 32

Facial, *8*
Fallopian tube, 143, *146*
Fascia lata, *54, 55*
Fasciectomy, 50
Febrile, 59, 61
Femoral, *8*
Femoral blood vessels, *89, 90*
Femoral nerve, *76*
Femur, *44, 46, 108*
Fibroblast, 65
Fibrosarcoma, 63
Fibula, *44, 46*
Fimbria(e), 146
Flexor carpi radialis muscle, *54*
Flexor carpi ulnaris muscle, *54*
Flexor digitorum longus muscle, *54*
Flexor digitorum superficialis muscle, *54*
Fontanelle(s), 177
Fornix of vagina, *147*
Fossa, 186
Fovea of eye, *70*
Frenzy, 182
Frontal, *8*
Frontal bone, *44*
Frontalis muscle, *54*
Fundus, 185
    of gall bladder, *110*
    of uterus, *146, 147*
Fungus, 197

Galactosemia, 140
Galaxy, 137
Gall bladder, 107, *108, 110*
Gamete(s), 143
Gametogenesis, 187
Ganglion(a), 97
Gastric, 185
Gastric artery, *89*
Gastritis, 176
Gastroclysis, 123, 188
Gastrocnemius muscle, *54, 55*, 187
Gastroenteritis, 176

Gastroenterology, 176
Gastrointestinal, 91
Gastronomical, 109
Gastropathy, 98
Gastroplegia, 112
Gastroscopy, 24
Genetic, 79
Genital, 143
Genitourinary, 176
Genuflect, 12
Geometry, 20
Geriatrics, 160, 162
Gerontology, 160
Gestation, 26
Gingivitis, 107
Glans, *148*
Glaucoma, 165, 176
Glomerulus, *144*
Glossolalia, 107
Glottis, 99
Glucose, 187
Gluteal, *10*
Gluteus maximus muscle, *55*
Gluteus medius muscle, *54*, 93
Glycolysis, 137, 140
Goiter, 176, 178
Gonad(s), 143
Gonadal artery, *89*
Gonadotropic, 103, 106
Gonadotropin, 187
Gonococcal, 176
Gracilis muscle, *54, 55*
Gracious, 20
Greek language, 145
Gustatory, 26, 28
Gynecogenic, 151
Gynecologist, 98
Gynecology, 98, 176
Gynecomastia, 151

Halitosis, 20
Hallux, *8*
Halogen, 137
Heart, *80, 81, 108, 128*
Hectare, 171
Hemangioma, 85
Hematemesis, 176
Hematologic, 92
Hematological, 65
Hematology, 176
Hematoma, 83, 86, 99, 176
Hematopoiesis, 24, 85, 95
Hematuria, 59, 61, 85, 97, 158, 176
Hemianopia, 95
Hemicranial, 182
Hemipelvectomy, 63
Hemiplegia, 35, 59, 61, 173
Hemiplegic, 3
Hemisphere, 32, 172
Hemolysis, 58, 187
Hemolytic, 176
Hemophilia, 3, 78, 102
Hemophiliac, 78
Hemorrhage, 59, 84